Research Ethics for Environmental Health

Research Ethics for Environmental Health explores the ethical basis of environmental health research and related aspects of risk assessment and control.

Environmental health encompasses the assessment and control of those environmental factors that can potentially affect human health, such as radiation, toxic chemicals and other hazardous agents. It is often assumed that the assessment part is just a matter of scientific research, and that control is a matter of implementing standards that unambiguously follow from that research. But it is less commonly understood that environmental health also requires addressing questions of an ethical nature. Coming from multiple disciplines and nine different countries, the contributors to this book critically examine a diverse range of ethical concerns in modern environmental health research.

This book will be of great interest to scholars and practitioners of environmental health, as well as researchers in applied ethics, environmental ethics, medical ethics, bioethics and those concerned with chemical and radiation protection.

Friedo Zölzer is professor of environmental sciences at the Faculty of Health and Social Sciences at the University of South Bohemia in Ceske Budejovice, Czech Republic. His main professional interests are radiological protection and environmental health, as well as related questions of ethics.

Gaston Meskens is a scientist, philosopher and artist. He works part-time with the Centre for Ethics and Value Inquiry of the Faculty of Arts and Philosophy of the University of Ghent, Belgium, and with the Science and Technology Studies group of the Belgian Nuclear Research Centre SCK•CEN.

Routledge Studies in Environment and Health

The study of the impact of environmental change on human health has rapidly gained momentum in recent years, and an increasing number of scholars are now turning their attention to this issue. Reflecting the development of this emerging body of work, the *Routledge Studies in Environment and Health* series is dedicated to supporting this growing area with cutting edge interdisciplinary research targeted at a global audience. The books in this series cover key issues such as climate change, urbanisation, waste management, water quality, environmental degradation and pollution, and examine the ways in which these factors impact human health from a social, economic and political perspective.

Comprising edited collections, co-authored volumes and single author monographs, this innovative series provides an invaluable resource for advanced undergraduate and postgraduate students, scholars, policy makers and practitioners with an interest in this new and important field of study.

Climate Change and Urban Health
The Case of Hong Kong as a Subtropical City
Emily Ying Yang Chan

Environmental Health and the U.S. Federal System
Sustainably Managing Health Hazards
Michael R. Greenberg and Dona Schneider

The Politics of the Climate Change–Health Nexus
Maximilian Jungmann

Research Ethics for Environmental Health
Edited by Friedo Zölzer and Gaston Meskens

For more information about this series, please visit: https://www.routledge.com/Routledge-Studies-in-Environment-and-Health/book-series/RSEH

Research Ethics for Environmental Health

Edited by
Friedo Zölzer and Gaston Meskens

Routledge
Taylor & Francis Group
LONDON AND NEW YORK

earthscan
from Routledge

First published 2022
by Routledge
2 Park Square, Milton Park, Abingdon, Oxon OX14 4RN

and by Routledge
605 Third Avenue, New York, NY 10158

Routledge is an imprint of the Taylor & Francis Group, an informa business

British Library Cataloguing-in-Publication Data
A catalogue record for this book is available from the British Library

Library of Congress Cataloging-in-Publication Data
A catalog record has been requested for this book

ISBN: 978-0-367-33203-7 (hbk)
ISBN: 978-1-032-17183-8 (pbk)
ISBN: 978-0-429-31843-6 (ebk)

DOI: 10.4324/9780429318436

Typeset in Bembo
by codeMantra

Contents

Figures

Tables

Contributors

Tom Børsen is an associate professor in techno-anthropology at Aalborg University, Denmark. His research clusters around different aspects of Responsible Technological Innovation, among them Ethical Technology Assessment and Interdisciplinary Policy Advice on Technological Risks.

Elisabeth Cardis is research professor in radiation epidemiology and head of the Radiation Programme at ISGlobal, Barcelona, Spain. Her main research area is epidemiology of radiation.

Carl F. Cranor is distinguished professor of philosophy and faculty member of the Environmental Toxicology Graduate Program at the University of California, Riverside, USA. His publications include *Legally Poisoned: How the Law Puts Us at Risk from Toxicants* (Harvard, 2011).

Kevin C. Elliott is professor of philosophy at Michigan State University, USA. His publications include *Is a Little Pollution Good for You? Incorporating Societal Values in Environmental Research* (Oxford, 2011) and *A Tapestry of Values: An Introduction to Values in Science* (Oxford, 2017).

Steven G. Gilbert is affiliate professor at the Department of Environmental and Occupational Health Sciences, University of Washington, Seattle, WA. His book, *A Small Dose of Toxicology - The Health Effects of Common Chemicals* was published in 2004 and will be a free e-book in 2021.

Chieko Kurihara is specially appointed professor at Kanagawa Dental University, and senior researcher/vice-chair of the Certified Review Board at the National Institutes for Quantum and Radiological Science and Technology, Japan. Her area of interest is bioethics and research ethics.

Liudmila Liutsko is postdoctoral fellow in the radiation program at ISGlobal, Barcelona, Spain. Her specializations are in mathematics, radioecology and psychology. She holds an MSc in environmental science and policy and a PhD in psychology.

Jacques Lochard is professor at the University of Nagasaki, Japan. Previously, he served as director of CEPN, an advisory institution in the field of radiation protection, in Fontenay-aux-Roses, France. He was also vice-chair of the International Commission on Radiological Protection (ICRP).

Gaston Meskens is a scientist, philosopher and artist. He works part-time with the Centre for Ethics and Value Inquiry of the Faculty of Arts and Philosophy of the University of Ghent, Belgium, and with the Science and Technology Studies group of the Belgian Nuclear Research Centre SCK•CEN.

Deborah Oughton is research director of the Centre for Environmental Radioactivity (CERAD) at the Norwegian University of Life Sciences. She has worked extensively on ethical and social aspects of radiation risk management.

Susana Paixao is professor of environmental health at the Polytechnic Institute of Coimbra, Portugal. She also serves as coordinator of the Health and Environment Center of the Academic Network of Health Sciences of Lusofonia and as the president of the International Federation of Environmental Health.

Colin L. Soskolne, professor emeritus, University of Alberta, Canada, is an occupational and environmental epidemiologist. A global leader in ethics for the profession, he received the International Society for Environmental Epidemiology 2021 Research Integrity Award.

Per Wikman-Svahn, is a researcher at the Division of Philosophy at the Royal Institute of Technology (KTH) in Stockholm, Sweden, where he does research and teaching on the philosophy of risk and uncertainty, philosophy of science and research ethics.

Friedo Zölzer is professor of environmental sciences in the Faculty of Health and Social Sciences at the University of South Bohemia in Ceske Budejovice, Czech Republic. His main professional interests are radiological protection and environmental health, as well as related questions of ethics.

Introduction

Gaston Meskens and Friedo Zölzer

Whatever may still happen after we have written and published these words, the year 2020 will be remembered as the beginning of a new reality for the theory and practice of environmental health. In that year, the outbreak of the SARS-CoV-2 virus has led to a global pandemic, followed by a worldwide mobilisation to control the spread of the virus, to protect the vulnerable and care for those who were affected by the Covid-19 disease and, last but not least, to develop medicines and vaccines that would allow the world to return to some form of normal life. Wherever we live on earth, and whatever our social context or professional background, every aspect of our daily life became determined by our individual and collective attempts to get control over the situation and to live with it. While a pandemic needs prompt practical and coordinated action, it also provides us with food for thought for the longer term about the world we live in. In that perspective, we see two reasons why this pandemic can be called a historical turning point in global environmental health governance.

First of all, any long-term thinking in the interest of controlling similar threats in the future logically needs to centre around the question of why and how a pandemic of this proportion and complex character could become possible. Already now, science has a simple answer to that question: it suggests that in many aspects the crisis is a direct consequence of the deplorable state into which humans themselves have brought their planet. This was already stated at the beginning of the outbreak (Vidal, 2020) and reiterated many times afterwards. An out-of-control globalised market and related industrial activities, in combination with a progressive destruction of natural habitats and loss of biodiversity, have set the conditions for the virus to emerge and spread. We know other global environmental health issues such as climate change or ocean acidification originate from the same general cause, but their threat to our health remains less 'visible' and 'tangible' as compared to how the SARS-CoV-2 virus directly affects the physical and psychological health of individual human beings. While it was said that 'the virus does not discriminate,' it became obvious very quickly that not everyone is affected in the same way and to the same extent. In addition to the common-sense

DOI: 10.4324/9780429318436-1

knowledge that the elderly and people with existing chronic conditions or compromised immune systems are more likely to suffer from Covid-19 came the insight that also the poor are more vulnerable. The SARS-CoV-2 virus threat became a complex problem among and closely interlinked with the other complex social and environmental problems that humanity is confronted with.

The second reason this pandemic can be called a turning point for global environmental health governance is to be found in the way it can be interpreted in the interest of fair and effective health risk governance. Three aspects need to be highlighted here:

1   Never before has the balance between freedom and responsibility in our own behaviour presented itself with such a tension on the level of the individual human being and hence for every one of us. That tension puts pressure on us and renders us insecure, anxious or defeatist. The freedom at stake is the freedom to enjoy life as we used to do in normal times. The responsibility charged upon us is our personal behaviour aimed at minimising the risk to become infected and consequently the risk to infect others. That responsibility is twofold and indivisible: our behaviour determines the risk not only to our own health but also that of those around us. We might not worry about our own health risk, but then we will always still put others in danger, including those we love and care about.

2   Never before has science, in its role of policy adviser, struggled so intensely with scientific uncertainty. Since the beginning of the emergence and spreading of the virus, experts have been solicited for urgent analysis of the situation and its evolution. Scientific data and insights into natural and social phenomena and with respect to possible cures are asked to be clear, factual and unambiguous, so as to enable politicians to quickly and easily translate analysis into policy recommendations and policy measures. By now, we know that such a demand is plainly unrealistic. Phenomena such as the behaviour of the virus and the reaction of our body and psyche to it, our social behaviour as a group facing a collective risk and, last but not least, the effectiveness and possible long-term side effects of vaccines will be better understood in the future, but the first phases of the pandemic have taught us that science, policy and society needed to heavily rely on precautionary measures only fragmentarily and vaguely supported by scientific insight and data. Some precautionary measures, such as special protection of the vulnerable, benefited from wide support, while others, such as lockdowns and curfews, have been defended as well as contested on both rational and ethical grounds. Whether as politician, epidemiologist, medical doctor, care worker or citizen, what we learned (or what we were reminded of) is that management of an acute crisis of this kind is short-term management that cannot but deal with the impossibility of calculable predictions.

3   Never before have we lived with a risk of which the assessment polarises and divides society to such an extent both in our local circles as well as on a world scale. The vision that, in order to control the virus in the longer term, only precautionary lockdown measures will do the job stands opposite to the vision that first and foremost we need to build up group immunity among the healthy population. Also the relevance, effectiveness and potential adverse effects of vaccines and vaccine campaigns have now become subject of societal debate on a scale never seen before. As a result, even interpretation of hands-on scientific data translatable into policy recommendations, such as the number of infections or the degree of hospital intensive care occupation, can still instigate divergent or even conflicting opinions on what is happening and on what to do. In addition, the idea of 'solidarity' gained new meaning and application. Citizens who organise or attend parties while society is in lockdown or who spend holidays abroad when there is the risk of bringing the virus home are generally considered not solidary with the rest of the population that wants to refrain from doing so in the general interest. Rich countries buying up vaccine stocks are considered not solidary with developing countries that work with more limited budgets and that face harder logistic challenges when it comes to distributing vaccines and deploying vaccination strategies.

The societal debate on how to cope with the virus, taking into account scientific uncertainties, ethical values, deliberate opinions, cowboy stories and conspiracy theories, continues and will continue for a time to come. It occurs on social media, within families, in labs, in schools, in offices and in hospitals, and in the fora, meeting rooms and corridors of political and economic powers. While that is a good thing as such, more and more citizens and civil society representatives have become frustrated with the fact that their opinion was not heard, let alone taken seriously. In a crisis that affects all of us personally in various ways and degrees, urgency cannot be used by authorities as an excuse to ignore the voices of the people, especially not in a post-emergency phase where acquired knowledge and insight can still diverge opinions on what to do next. The only way to gain support for policy measures in that situation is by simply deliberating with those affected by these measures.

Meanwhile, life continues, and the need for concern about other aspects of environmental health remains. The seeds of this publication were planted at the Fourth International Symposium on Ethics of Environmental Health that took place in Budweis, Czech Republic, in September 2018. That means most of the contributions to this book were written before the outbreak of the SARS-CoV-2 virus; although it is possible to see these contributions in a 'new light' given the changed situation, their focus and elaboration of reasoning and their recommendations obviously remain as valid and accurate as before.

This selection of papers from the Fourth Budweis Symposium follows two earlier publications which contained contributions to the Second and Third

Symposia held in 2014 and 2016, respectively. Both of these were published by Routledge as part of their series 'Studies in Environment and Health', the first one addressing some fundamental issues of 'Ethics of Environmental Health' (Zölzer and Meskens, 2017), the second one more specifically 'Environmental Health Risks – Ethical Aspects' (Zölzer and Meskens, 2019). Like the earlier volumes, the current one contains 12 chapters arranged in four sections. The first three contributions throw light on the global context in which questions of environmental health have to be necessarily addressed two decades into the twenty-first century. The second and third group of chapters focus on questions of toxicology research (with particular emphasis on possible conflicts of interest) and radiological protection (with particular emphasis on stakeholder involvement). The last three contributions address questions of research ethics in a more general way, discussing underlying social values and ethical principles.

We would like to express our deep gratitude to all our co-authors who carried this project through in spite of all the difficulties they and their families as well as their institutions have been facing since we first invited them to contribute to this book. The same is true for the reviewers who took a real interest in ensuring the quality of the individual chapters, over and beyond a formal approval of their suitability for publication. And finally, we would like to thank the electricity provider for the region of South Bohemia, E.ON, as well as the University of South Bohemia in Budweis for financial and organisational support, without which the Fourth International Symposium on Ethics of Environmental Health would probably not have been possible.

References

Vidal, John. 2020. 'Destroyed Habitat Creates the Perfect Conditions for Coronavirus to Emerge'. *Scientific American*. March 18, 2020. https://www.scientificamerican.com/article/destroyed-habitat-creates-the-perfect-conditions-for-coronavirus-to-emerge/
Zölzer, Friedo, and Gaston Meskens, eds. 2017. *Ethics of Environmental Health*. Routledge, UK. http://hdl.handle.net/1854/LU-8555283.
———, eds. 2019. *Environmental Health Risks: Ethical Aspects*. 1st edition. Routledge, UK.

Part 1

Environmental health ethics in general

1 Environmental health in a global context

Susana Paixao

The origin of *environmental health* happened because of the need to create a balance in the relationship between humankind and environment (Ribeiro, 2004). According to the World Health Organization (WHO), *environmental health* addresses all physical, chemical and biological factors external to a person that affect health and well-being. It thus includes the assessment and control of environmental factors that may affect health. It is intended to prevent disease and to create health-friendly environments.

In recent decades, humanity has transformed natural resources and ecosystems with a speed and extent never known before in history. Urbanization, population growth and economic growth have led to a complex environmental situation in which poor air quality, declining drinking water sources, soil and food contamination, and climate and environmental change are blended beyond the equilibrium capacities of ecosystems and individuals to maintain themselves (Soares da Silva, 2013).

In National Geographic, which has been paying particular attention to environmental issues globally, we can see several examples showing that something is happening with the environment in which we live and that our actions are severely degrading existing natural resources. Examples include the Aral Sea, between Kazakhstan and Uzbekistan, which was one of the four largest lakes in the world. After decades of serving to water cotton fields, it has almost disappeared! Or, the case of the Alaska Glacier Columbia, which flows directly into the sea and was roughly in the same position from 1794 (the year it was discovered) until 1980 and, as of 2014, that is within 18 years, the nose of the glacier retracted about 19 km, thus being one of the fastest disappearing glaciers in the world; or, Shanghai's growth, and the theft of land for Dubai to grow, and the deforestation of the Amazon rainforest, are some of the many examples of what is going on in the world that are compromising the health and well-being of the world population.

Health and *environment* have always been closely related. However, a variation in the importance given to their relationship has been noted over time. It is considered that the first allusion to this relationship was made by Hippocrates. In his treatise 'On air, water and places' he talks of 'fully recognizing the value of the principle of geographical conditions and climate influences

DOI: 10.4324/9780429318436-3

on health'. In the nineteenth century, John Snow, pioneer in spatial epidemiology, discovered in 1854 that the epidemic of cholera that ravaged London was transmitted by water, a fundamental discovery that would subsequently control the spread of the disease. Already in the twentieth century in 1951, in Japan, pollution as a cause of disease was first highlighted in the city of Minamata. This serious disease, called Minamata disease, whose symptoms are mainly a weakening of the muscles that can go in extreme cases to madness, paralysis, coma and death in the following weeks, is caused by the release of methyl mercury into the water, causing mercury poisoning in people who consume the fish taken from this water. It is the first documented such study of the health impacts of the environment.

We consider that *environmental health* was elevated to a higher level with the publication of 'Silent Spring' by Rachel Carson. She focused on how DDT (dichlorodiphenyltrichloroethane), an organochlorine pesticide, enters the food chain and how it can affect not only birds, but also humans, establishing a clear relationship between the environment and the health of people exposed to a specific substance. DDT was the first modern pesticide widely used during and after World War II to combat mosquito vectors of diseases such as malaria and dengue.

But it has probably been with the 'Love Canal' case in the United States and 'Chernobyl' in Europe that the relationship between *health* and *environment* has become so evident and resulted in concrete actions, particularly in the Western world.

The Love Canal case occurred in the United States of America in a neighbourhood near Niagara Falls, New York, where, in the 1940s, a chemical company disposed of tons of chemical by-products onto lands over which in 1953 a school was built and a whole neighbourhood, where after an exceptionally rainy year in 1962, the chemicals started coming to the surface causing serious health problems in the local residents.

This case attracted national attention, and it was the genesis of the Superfund, a U.S. federal government programme designed to fund the clean-up of sites contaminated with hazardous substances and pollutants.

In 1986, a nuclear reactor exploded in the Chernobyl Nuclear Power Station, which is located near the city of Pripyat in the Ukraine. The radioactive cloud that formed after the disaster affected almost all of the countries in Europe. The world realized that the existence of borders did not protect from environmental contamination.

As a result of the Chernobyl catastrophe, European countries initiated the first-ever process to eliminate the most significant environmental threats to human health. Progress towards this goal has been driven by a series of ministerial conferences held every five years coordinated by WHO/Europe. These environment and health conferences are unique, bringing together different sectors to shape European policies and actions on environment and health. The first conference was held in Frankfurt in 1989. We can highlight the

Fifth Conference held in Parma, Italy, on March 2010 that resulted in The Parma Declaration, the first time-limited outcome of the *environment* and *health* process. Governments of the 53 European member-states set clear targets to reduce the adverse health impacts of environmental threats in the next decade. As important was the Sixth Ministerial Conference on Environment and Health held in Ostrava Czech Republic in June 2017, and 'The Ostrava Declaration' was introduced with the motto 'Better Health. Better Environment. Sustainable Choices'. This defined four goals:

1   Leverage the European environment and health process to achieve selected Sustainable Development Goals;
2   Addresses the 'unfinished business' of environment and health in Europe;
3   Promote coherence across all policy levels and establish inclusive platforms for dialogue; and
4   Develop national portfolios for action and strong intersectorial coordination.

To better achieve these goals, the WHO/Europe published a second assessment report on 'Environmental health inequalities in Europe' (2019), which considers the distribution of environmental risks and injuries within countries and shows that unequal environmental conditions, exposure risks and related health outcomes affect citizens daily in all settings where people live, work and spend their time. The report documents the magnitude of environmental health inequalities within countries through 19 inequality indicators on urban housing and working conditions, basic services and injuries. This report highlights that inequalities in risks and outcomes occur in all countries in the WHO European region. The latest evidence confirms that socially disadvantaged population subgroups are those most affected by environmental hazards, causing avoidable health effects and contributing to health inequalities.

At the Ostrava meeting, delegates agreed on the importance of addressing the need to accelerate progress on health and environment and, in particular, to address the environment-related health goals and targets of the 2030 Sustainable Development Agenda.

There are as many as 17 Sustainable Development Goals. They were adopted on 25 September 2015 in a way to address poverty, protect the planet and assure prosperity for all. All of the goals are interconnected; we highlight goal number 3 'Good Health and Well-being' to ensure healthy lives and promote well-being for all at all ages. It is my conviction that this goal must be at the centre of all the other goals.

The WHO provides a panorama of objectives that must be taken into account. Nine facts for preventing disease are highlighted relating to healthy environments because today about one in four deaths across the globe are due to environmental factors and, according to the WHO, every year an estimated 12.6 million people die as a result of living or working in an unhealthy environment.

More than 100 diseases and injuries are related to environmental risk factors, such as air, water and soil pollution, chemical exposures, climate change and ultraviolet radiation. But there are also positive indicators – such as the number of deaths from infectious diseases such as diarrhoea and malaria, which are often related to poor water, sanitation and waste management – that have declined. This happened because of the improvements to basic sanitation such as the increases in access to safe water and sanitation alongside better access to immunization, insecticide-treated mosquito nets and essential medicines. But, despite all efforts to achieve better health among populations, it is important to highlight counter-current movements such as anti-vaccination groups. The measles example, a disease which had been declared eradicated in most European countries, saw cases reappearing in large numbers due to misinformed populations.

The WHO also highlights the relationship between the vulnerability to environmental-related diseases and the age of the population, emphasizing the fact that younger children and older people are most affected by these diseases. Annually, 1.7 million deaths in children under 5 years of age are attributable to the environment. The most prominent causes of death are lower respiratory tract infections, such as pneumonia, and diarrheal diseases. And 4.9 million deaths in adults between 50 and 75 years of age are attributable to the environment. Unlike children under 5, older adults are most affected by non-communicable diseases. It is also important take into account that environmental impacts are uneven across different social groups, not only by their social status, income, employment and education but also by noneconomic aspects such as age, gender and ethnicity.

Also the geographical place where people are born and live, as reported by WHO, helps to establish a relationship between environmental issues and the health of populations. Thus, low- and middle-income countries in the WHO Southeast Asia and Western Pacific regions had the largest environmentally related disease burden in 2012, with a total of 7.3 million deaths, most attributable to indoor and outdoor air pollution. But, at the same time, WHO with its stakeholders are working on prevention; they highlight the importance of the health and other sectors needing to work together to reduce the environmental burden of disease, such as reducing traffic congestion and improving public transport networks as important determinants of air pollution, and usually require cooperation with the transport sector and city planners. Because of this, it is important that local governance address environmental health planning. Municipalities are natural leaders of the local environment and health planning. They are often involved in developing the local economy, including transport, tourism and industry, and can play an important role in health planning if they are aware of the potential risks and benefits and are provided with the tools and support they need.

It is therefore increasingly important to pay attention to this phenomenon as the United Nations estimates that 66% of the world's population will live in cities by 2050 and, according to James Canton (2011), by 2040, most of the world's population will be living in megacities, cities containing at least 10 million people.

According to the World Bank (2015), town planning is important for understanding the maxim 'think globally, act locally'. Urban management and development highly impacts the surrounding environment. The ways in which this is implemented are vital to the health of the environment. Corporations need to be aware of global communities when expanding their companies to new locations. Not only do corporations need to be aware of global differences, but they must also pay closer attention to urban and rural areas that plan on expanding or changing the dynamics of their communities. As stated by the World Bank (2015),

> addressing the complex urban environmental problems, in order to improve urban livability through Urban Environmental Strategies, involves taking stock of the existing urban environmental problems, their comparative analysis and prioritization, setting out objectives and targets, and identification of various measures to meet these objectives.

The concept of a 'circular city' or a 'circular city-region' derives from the circular economy model applied in the spatial territorial dimension. It can be associated with the concept of a 'self-sustainable' regenerative city, as discussed by Zeleny (2010).

As the Ellen MacArthur Foundation mentioned at the report 'CE100 Circularity in the Built Environment' (2016), the circular economy model has been defined as an economic model which is 'regenerative by design', with the aim to retain as much value as possible of products, parts and materials, focusing on the lifecycle of materials to 'close-the-loop' by recovering all wastes as a resource for new productive cycles.

So cities must increasingly become circular cities and leave the concept of linear cities (take, make, leave). The circular city view should take into account the built environment, the energy system, urban mobility systems and the creation of an urban bioeconomy. Obviously, this transition cannot happen without a fundamental change in behaviour and thinking. Using without being a consumer or sharing rather than accumulating are the new (and old) ways of being in the world and the basis for building a circular economy in which society is the central focus without compromising resources that future generations will need.

All of this is becoming increasingly important as predictions state that the trend is for an ever-increasing footprint. Hence, the importance of taking action now.

Climate change has been identified as one of the greatest environmental, social and economic threats facing the planet and humanity today. Climate change impacts health both directly, as storm, drought, flood, heatwave, temperature change and wildfires, and indirectly, such as water and air quality, excessive land use and ecological changes, but is strongly mediated by environmental, social and public health determinants.

The United Nations Framework Convention on Climate Change (UNFCCC) and the ongoing negotiations on the climate regime have as their long-term objective the stabilization of greenhouse gas (GHG) concentrations in the atmosphere to a level that avoids dangerous anthropogenic interference with the climate system. To achieve this objective, the average annual global land surface temperature should not exceed 2°C above pre-industrial levels.

GHG emissions are a common phenomenon across sectors of activity, thus justifying the cross-cutting nature of climate change mitigation and adaptation policies.

Indeed, to address the problem of climate change there are essentially two lines of action – mitigation and adaptation. While mitigation is the process that aims to reduce GHG emissions into the atmosphere, adaptation is the process that seeks to minimize the negative effects of climate change impacts on biophysical and socioeconomic systems.

Climate change affects social and environmental determinants of health – clean air, safe drinking water, sufficient food and secure shelter – and brings many risks to the world's population such as extreme heat, natural disasters and variable rainfall patterns.

Extreme air temperatures directly contribute to deaths from cardiovascular and respiratory diseases, especially among the elderly. High temperatures increase the levels of both ozone and other air pollutants that aggravate cardiovascular and respiratory disease and pollen and other aeroallergens.

Globally, the number of reported weather-related natural disasters, according to the Intergovernmental Panel on Climate Change (IPCC, 2018), has more than tripled since the 1960s. Every year, these disasters result in over 60,000 deaths, mainly in developing countries.

WHO, in its 'COP24 Special Report: Health and Climate Change' (2018) states that rising sea levels and increasingly extreme weather events will destroy homes, medical facilities and other essential services. More than half of the world's population lives within 60 km of the sea. 'People may be forced to move, which in turn heightens the risk of a range of health effects, from mental disorders to communicable diseases.'

Increasingly variable rainfall patterns are likely to affect the supply of fresh water. And, according to the same report, lack of safe water can compromise hygiene and increase the risk of diarrheal disease. Floods are also increasing in frequency and intensity, and the frequency and intensity of extreme precipitation is expected to continue to increase throughout the century. Floods contaminate freshwater supplies, heighten the risk of water-borne diseases and create breeding grounds for disease-carrying insects such as mosquitoes. They also cause drownings and physical injuries, damage homes and disrupt the supply of medical and health services. Rising temperatures and variable precipitation are likely to decrease the production of staple foods in many of the poorest regions. Furthermore, climatic conditions strongly affect water-borne diseases and diseases transmitted through insects, snails or other cold-blooded animals. Changes in climate can lengthen the transmission season of certain vector-borne diseases and expand their geographic range. Malaria, caused by *Aedes aegypti* mosquito (vector of dengue and yellow fever), among others, is strongly influenced by climate.

All populations will be affected by climate change, but some are more vulnerable than others. People living in small island developing states and other coastal regions, megacities and mountainous and polar regions are particularly vulnerable.

The IPCC report, 'Global warming at 1.5°C' (2018), describes the large difference between the impacts of temperature increases of +1.5°C and +2°C and points out that the alternative can only be a massive reduction in the use of fossil fuels and concomitantly in greenhouse gas emissions, which would require us to 'apply rapid, comprehensive and unprecedented changes in all aspects of society.'

The 2030 Agenda for Sustainable Development and its Sustainable Development Goals (SDGs) reflect the common understanding that a healthy environment is integral to the full enjoyment of basic human rights, including the rights to life, health, food, water and sanitation. Directly tackling the interlinkages between environment and human health presents new and interwoven opportunities to meet the SDGs in a more cost-effective and beneficial manner. To 'ensure healthy lives and promote well-being for all at all ages' (SDG3) – which includes a specific target related to air quality – cannot be achieved over the long term without explicit action on terrestrial ecosystems (SDG15), oceans (SDG14), cities (SDG11), water and sanitation (SDG6).

Air pollution is the world's largest single environmental risk to health. According to WHO, as much as 7 million people across the world die each year due to everyday exposure to poor air quality. But it cannot be viewed in isolation. The zoonotic diseases like, Zika, West Nile virus or Ebola, among others, spread from animals to humans and are currently emerging every four months, with the main drivers being exponential population growth, intensive livestock breeding (there are 36 billion domestic animals on the planet) and concomitant disturbed environments and biodiversity loss. Strengthening healthy ecosystems is key to preventing or slowing the emergence of these costly diseases.

The new approach 'One Health', as mentioned by CDC (Centers for Disease Control and Prevention, 2017),

> recognizes that the health of people is connected to the health of animals and the environment. It is a collaborative, multisectorial, and transdisciplinary approach – working at the local, regional, national, and global levels – with the goal of achieving optimal health outcomes recognizing the interconnection between people, animals, plants, and their shared environment. A One Health approach is important because 6 out of every 10 infectious diseases in humans are spread from animals.

In conclusion, the area of health and environment is part of the group of major areas of study/academic areas within the health sciences. This area is still growing but has proved to be fundamental to societal development. All human action has an impact on nature – positive or negative. The intensity and nature of this impact is commensurate with social organization and human-developed economic activities. Among the problems presented by this relationship between humans and nature, those relating to the environment and which focus on health, stand out. The scope of environmental health in public health is extremely broad and involves serious issues such as global warming, ozone depletion, natural disasters, vector proliferation, housing conditions and basic sanitation, among many other health- and environment-related factors. In order to contextualize health–environment relationships, it is necessary to understand the evolution of environmental issues in the daily lives of communities. It is also important to understand their magnitude, seeking to identify at the local level the various positive and negative relationships between people and the environment that permeates them; the introduction of policies and initiatives aimed at detecting risk situations as well as actions to be taken to solve problems are needed.

It is also important to highlight the environmental health workforce. The professionals in this area of knowledge make sure our surrounding environments (our home, our workplace and the places that we visit and stay) are safe, hygienic and healthy, focusing on prevention. They easily access community assets, with a greater knowledge of local customs, familiarity of local risks, and with a superior command of local language, thus allowing people to act locally while thinking globally. Environmental health professionals are aware of the potential risks and benefits and are equipped with the tools and support needed to address environmental health challenges. In particular, as professionals they can save money and lives, promote health and wellness and protect the environment for future generations. Maintaining a healthy environment is central to increasing not only the quality of life but also the number of healthy years of life. It is the ethical duty of those in the public health field to work in the public interest to maintain and increase the quality of life as well as increase the number of healthy years of life. Other chapters in this volume address the ethical dimensions of environmental health.

Bibliography

Borghini A. 9th European Public Health Conference: Poster Displays. 2015;475.

Centers for Disease Control and Prevention. 'One Health'. 2017. Available online: https://www.cdc.gov/onehealth/ (accessed on 26 June 2019)

Custard B. 'Building the Future Environmental Health Workforce'. *J Environ Health* 2010;8(5):275.

Ellen MacArthur Foundation. CE100 Circularity in the Built Environment: Case Studies. A Compilation of Case Studies from the CE100. 2016. Available online: https://www.ellenmacarthurfoundation.org/assets/downloads/Built-Env-Co. Project.pdf (accessed on 26 June 2019).

Enriquez Collins A. 'What it means…'. *J Environ Health* 2014;76(9):6–9.

Fabian N. 'The future of environmental health'. *J Environ Health* 2013;76(5):70.

Fitzpatrick M, Bonnefoy X. *Environmental Health Services in Europe 3: professional profiles*. Geneva: World Health Organization. Regional Office for Europe. 1998.

Fitzpatrick M. *Environmental Health Services in Europe 6: the development of professional associations*. Geneva: World Health Organization. Regional Office for Europe. 2002.

Frumkin H. *Environmental Health: From Global to Local*. San Francisco: John Wiley. 2005.

Girardet, H. Regenerative Cities. In *Green Economy Reader. Studies in Ecological Economics*. Shmelev, S., Ed.; Springer: Cham, Switzerland, 2017; pp. 183–204.

Intergovernmental Panel on Climate Change (IPCC), 'Global Warming at 1.5°C'. 2018. Available from: https://www.ipcc.ch/sr15/ (accessed on 26 June 2019)

James C. 'The Extreme Future of Megacitie'. 2011. Available from: https://rss.onlinelibrary.wiley.com/doi/pdf/10.1111/j.1740-9713.2011.00485.x (accessed on 26 June 2019)

Jason W, Marie A. 'Trends in the Environmental Health Job Market for New Graduates'. *J Environ Health*. 2015;80(2).

Lourtie P, Rocha Pinto ML. *Adequação dos Cursos de Tecnologias da Saúde*. Relatório para o Ministério da Saúde. Lisboa: Ministério da Saúde; 2007.

Marion JW, Murphy TJ. 'A Fork in the Road for Environmental Health Workforce Development and US Public Health'. *J Environ Health*. 2016;79(2):40–43.

Mead L. UNEP, WHO Launch Partnership on Environmental Health [Internet]. 2018. Available from: http://sdg.iisd.org/news/unep-who-launch-partnership-on-environmental-health/ (accessed on 26 June 2019)

Musoke D, Ndejjo R, Atusingwize E, Halage AA. The Role of Environmental Health in One Health: A Uganda Perspective. *One Health* [Internet]. Elsevier B.V.; 2016; 2:157–160.

National Geographic. Available online: https://www.nationalgeographic.com/environment/climate-change/ (accessed on 26 June 2019)

Panis S, Araujo MO De, Verçoze MV, Brito JS. 'Educação ambiental: avaliação da abordagem não formal na escola municipal professor benjamim soares de carvalho teresina – PI'. *VII CONNEPI - Congresso Norte Nordeste de Pesquisa e Inovação*, 2012.

Ribeiro H. 'Saúde Pública e meio ambiente: evolução do conhecimento e da prática, alguns aspectos éticos'. Saúde e Sociedade; 2004; 3(1):70–80.

Robles SLRDE, Chavéz MGG, Ballesteros AC. 'The Environmental Health Field: An Opportunity to Reach Science Education Goals'. *Ambient Soc* [Internet]. 2015;18(4):73–92.

Schmidt L, Gil Nave J, Guerra J. *Educação Ambiental: Balanço e perspectivas para uma agenda mais sustentável*. Lisboa: Imprensa de Ciências Sociais; 2010.

Silva F, Bento A. 'Educação ambiental e cidadania: Os desafios da escola de hoje'. *Cadernos de Pesquisa*; 2002; 118:189–205.

United Nations. 'Transforming Our World: The 2030 Agenda for Sustainable Development'. 2015. Available online: https://www.un.org/ga/search/view_doc.asp?symbol=A/RES/70/1&Lang=E (accessed on 26 June 2019) (accessed on 26 June 2019)

United Nations Environment Program. 'Healthy Environment, Healthy People'. 2016. Available online: https://www.unenvironment.org/news-and-stories/story/healthy-environment-healthy-people (accessed on 26 June 2019)

Walker Jr. B. 'The Environmental Health Workforce'. 2009;72:38. Available online: http://www.ncbi.nlm.nih.gov/pubmed/19908437 (accessed on 26 June 2019)

World Bank. 'World Inclusive Cities Approach Paper'. 2015. Available online: http://documents.worldbank.org/curated/pt/402451468169453117/pdf/AUS8539-REVISED-WP-P148654-PUBLIC-Box393236B-Inclusive-Cities-Approach-Paper-w-Annexes-final.pdf (accessed on 26 June 2019)

World Health Organization. 'Ostrava Declaration'. 2017. Available online: http://www.euro.who.int/__data/assets/pdf_file/0007/341944/OstravaDeclaration_SIGNED.pdf?ua=1 (accessed on 26 June 2019)

World Health Organization. 'COP24 Special Report Health and Climate Change'. 2018. Available online: https://www.who.int/globalchange/publications/COP24-report-health-climate-change/en/ (accessed on 26 June 2019)

World Health Organization. 'Environmental Health Inequalities in Europe. Second Assessment Report'. 2019. Available online: http://www.euro.who.int/en/publications/abstracts/environmental-health-inequalities-in-europe-second-assessment-report-2019 (accessed on 26 June 2019)

Zeleny, M. Knowledge Management and Strategic Self-Sustainability: A Human Systems Perspective. In *Making Strategies in Spatial Planning*. Cerreta, M., Concilio, G., Monno, V., Eds.; Springer: Dordrecht, The Netherlands, 2010; pp. 257–280.

2 Values and ethics as upstream determinants of population health

The Earth Charter at the local level

Colin L. Soskolne

Introduction

The earliest warning from science about human activity causing damage to the climate system dates back to 1896. The article by Arrhenius (1896) addressed the problem of carbon dioxide emissions arising from the industrial revolution and accumulating in the upper atmosphere. Arrhenius noted consequences over the longer term of a greenhouse effect and thus was first among scientists to anticipate negative impacts on the climate system. Despite this, as well as the decades-later *Club of Rome Report* (Meadows et al., 1972), evidence continues to mount; humanity's trajectory augurs poorly for the ongoing flourishing – indeed, continuation – of life on Earth.

Three factors were revealed as root causes of a worsening trajectory of decline by Ehrlich and Holdren (1971) in their now famous identity; it was some 50 years ago that they first brought attention to the relationship between 'impacts' on the one hand, and 'population', 'affluence' and 'technology' on the other hand. Despite this important work, worsening trends have continued globally because of woefully inadequate attention paid by policymakers to questions these authors raise relating to the overriding negative dimensions of population, affluence and technology.

More recently, Soskolne and Bertollini (1999) led the production of a World Health Organization (WHO) Discussion Document on global ecological integrity as a cornerstone of public health. This document was the most accessed document on the WHO EURO website for three successive years, thus proving of significant advocacy importance in the sustainability movement. Yet worsening trends continue globally.

So much more has been written on the topic since the *Club of Rome Report*. Despite all of this work, carbon dioxide accumulations in the upper atmosphere continue unabated, with levels exceeding those considered safe for the sustainability of life (as we know it) on Earth.

Most recently, the *World Scientists' Warning to Humanity: A Second Notice* (Ripple et al., 2017) is meant to draw attention to both the magnitude and urgency of these matters. Despite such efforts, all warnings are going unheeded from a practical perspective at the highest levels of policy and influence, with

DOI: 10.4324/9780429318436-4

consequent continuing disruptions and declines in that which sustains life, along with accelerating species' extinctions (Butler, 2016; Ripple et al., 2017, 2020, 2021).

In McMichael's 1993 text, *Planetary Overload: Global Environmental Change and the Health of the Human Species* (McMichael, 1993), the importance of upstream determinants of health and well-being were brought starkly to the attention of public health professionals, and particularly to those in the core discipline of public health, namely those in epidemiology. Some 25 years later, the practical effect on policy of those who have taken up McMichael's challenge continues to be minimal at best, and the situation worsens.

Instead of remaining part of the problem, how could most scientists (indeed, most citizens) become part of the solution? How much more science is needed to inform policy in support of much-needed advocacy? Is it science alone that is needed to change the current trajectory, or are questions of values and ethics at least as relevant to a remedy? Are science, values and ethics tightly interwoven? These questions are addressed in this chapter.

Linear reductionism and wholism as paradigms in science

Most scientists have traditionally adhered to the paradigm of linear reductionism - single causes along linear paths for specific effects – and this paradigm has provided understandings of the physical world. While this approach has been paramount for the advancement of our knowledge of the physical world, the focus on linear reductionism to the relative exclusion of systems approaches (also known as wholism) has been a disservice to the advancement of explanations around complexity, regardless of the physical system(s) being investigated, however small or large. The problem has become systemic with universities structuring themselves as compartmentalized, disciplinary silos, each competing for limited resources in order to support economic growth.

Systems approaches in science, on the other hand, are integrative; they lean on multi-, inter- and trans-disciplinary methods to explain a phenomenon and, in so doing, they embrace complexity. Since most questions of sustainability are complex in nature, sustainability has not been served well by linear reductionism. While uni-, multi- and inter-disciplinary efforts have been fruitful in advancing knowledge, transdisciplinarity is an approach that facilitates thinking outside of the box (i.e., outside of existing and more dominant paradigms). In studying human health, transdisciplinarity integrates the natural, social and health sciences in a humanities context and, in so doing, transcends each of their traditional boundaries. Emergent concepts and methods are the hallmark of the transdisciplinary effort (Soskolne, 2003). To achieve transdisciplinarity, continued movement from the silo-based, compartmentalized approaches in our universities will be necessary to more effectively address problems of a complex nature, sustainability being one such problem.

It behooves us to consider influences that incentivize the adoption of one paradigmatic approach over another. Not only is the self-interest of the discipline at play, but external to science are other influences that drive the very nature of questions in science and the methods by which they are addressed. In addition to how questions are scientifically addressed, pressures and influences motivate what is and what is not given due attention. Biases of various kinds operate in science and the way these are handled has ethical implications. Incentives for and against thinking outside of the box are relevant to how the chosen paradigm plays out.

The interplay of interests, values and ethics as upstream determinants of health, and also of policy

Powerful interests, bent on maintaining the *status quo*, provide incentives usually of a direct or indirect financial nature, not only to scientists, but also to those in influential roles in government, to not think outside the box (Cranor 2011; Soskolne 2017, 2019). This is done specifically to protect special interests to which many in positions of power are beholden. Special interests include those in the corporate structure with their short-term reports to shareholders (profit-driven), as well as political leaders in (usually) four-year election cycles in many countries (power-driven).

When scientists do prevail, systematic unethical attacks on their evidence are made in order to suppress what could be, or on what may have been, discovered. In the sustainability realm, by virtue of these forces and distinct value differences, little to no action has resulted in policies that, if implemented, might have effected needed changes in humankind's trajectory (from a path of decline to one of sustainability).

While pressures to maintain the *status quo* dominate, new technologies and chemicals continue to be foisted into commerce (Cranor 2011) before being adequately tested for their ethical appropriateness or safety. These technologies and chemicals negatively impact people who are biologically susceptible and, even more critically, the very ecosystems that sustain all forms of life. The latter are degraded such that delicately balanced natural systems upon which humanity depends for the generation of fresh air, pure water and nutritious soils are reaching and, indeed, exceeding tipping points; their life-sustaining functions are being diminished, and even eliminated, placing the entire human enterprise – and life writ large – in grave jeopardy (Ripple et al., 2017, 2020, 2021).

Questions of how much time remains to change course, and by what mechanisms, are topics of ongoing assessment.

Moving towards change

To motivate change, we first need to see ourselves as being part of, and not separate from, the ecosystems within which we live. Such a reorientation will motivate us to engage in being part of the solution in seeking a path of sustainability rather than remaining detached and thus part of the problem of accelerating declines.

To reconnect people to their complete dependence on the ecosystems in which they live, new approaches are needed. An eco- and/or bio-centric worldview is essential if those anthropocentric human behaviours that contribute to maintaining the *status quo* are to change in favour of moving humanity onto a sustainable path. As proposed here, values and ethics are the levers of such change. Indeed, the values and ethical principles embodied in *The Earth Charter* were drafted to provide humanity with the motivation, framework and tools for effecting needed change. And these have been in place since 2000 (*The Earth Charter*, 2000).

Critical to understanding how change is possible, is recognizing that people will generally operate in their local context more so than in a global context. For instance, climate change, being a global phenomenon, is effectively addressed by individuals at the local level where they more likely would have a greater degree of control and influence. René Jules Dubos (Dubos, 1977) is credited for having made famous Jacques Ellul's environmental maxim: 'Think globally, act locally.'

It is at the local level where values and ethics must be applied. Top-down (global) and bottom-up (local) efforts are urgently needed if the path forward is to become one that is sustainable. Using the values and ethical principles of *The Earth Charter*, access to some examples is provided; they demonstrate how different local approaches to its implementation have been undertaken around the world.

The Earth Charter: Essentials

The Earth Charter was launched in 2000 to provide a set of universal values and ethical principles for people in whatever ecological circumstance they find themselves (*The Earth Charter*, 2000). Its purpose remains to shift humanity from its current trajectory of decline in all that sustains life on Earth to a path of sustainability.

The initial proposal for *The Earth Charter* was envisaged by Maurice Strong for the 1992 Earth Summit held in Rio de Janeiro. By 2000, under the co-stewardship of Strong and Mikhail Gorbachev, an international grassroots movement produced *The Earth Charter* as it exists today. As with any living document, fine-tuning may be warranted. However, there should be no need to reinvent the wheel. *The Earth Charter* provides our best hope for aligning values and ethical guidance in our personal lives as well as in all aspects of socioeconomic organization and governance.

The Earth Charter is a four-page soft law instrument containing universal values and principles brought together in an accessible document to save us from ourselves (*The Earth Charter*, 2000). In summary, it is structured as follows:

- **PREAMBLE** (values followed by four first-order principles)
  - Respect and care for the community of life
  - Ecological integrity

- Social and economic justice
- Democracy, nonviolence and peace

- **THE WAY FORWARD** (commitment to *The Earth Charter's* values)

The Earth Charter is accessible in some 65 different languages. The four first-order ethical principles identify the four domains of focus, providing within each domain the second-order ethical principles which speak to ethical duties for their implementation, as follows:

I   Respect and Care for the Community of Life
   - Respect Earth and life in all its diversity.
   - Care for the community of life with understanding, compassion and love.
   - Build democratic societies that are just, participatory, sustainable and peaceful.
   - Secure Earth's bounty and beauty for present and future generations.
II Ecological Integrity
   - Protect and restore the integrity of Earth's ecological systems, with special concern for biological diversity and the natural processes that sustain life.
   - Prevent harm as the best method of environmental protection and, when knowledge is limited, apply a precautionary approach.
   - Adopt patterns of production, consumption and reproduction that safeguard Earth's regenerative capacities, human rights and community well-being.
   - Advance the study of ecological sustainability and promote the open exchange and wide application of the knowledge acquired.
III Social and Economic Justice
   - Eradicate poverty as an ethical, social and environmental imperative.
   - Ensure that economic activities and institutions at all levels promote human development in an equitable and sustainable manner.
   - Affirm gender equality and equity as prerequisites to sustainable development and ensure universal access to education, healthcare and economic opportunity.
   - Uphold the right of all, without discrimination, to a natural and social environment supportive of human dignity, bodily health and spiritual well-being, with special attention to the rights of indigenous peoples and minorities.
IV Democracy, Nonviolence and Peace
   - Strengthen democratic institutions at all levels and provide transparency and accountability in governance, inclusive participation in decision-making, and access to justice.
   - Integrate into formal education and life-long learning the knowledge, values and skills needed for a sustainable way of life.
   - Treat all living beings with respect and consideration.
   - Promote a culture of tolerance, nonviolence and peace.

Examples of *The Earth Charter's* implementation/adoption

In addition to the thousands of endorsements representing millions of people, *The Earth Charter* is endorsed by industries, governments at various levels, United Nations (UN) agencies, nongovernmental organizations (NGOs) and religious groups (*The Earth Charter*, 2019). It is not the purpose of this chapter to discuss the merits or extent of endorsements, but rather to focus on larger-scale initiatives that have embraced and, indeed, advanced *The Earth Charter*.

Six examples of *The Earth Charter* forming the anchor for collective thought and action around the world follow below. The article title is used to highlight the initiative; online access to each is provided under the reference list at the end. The title is indicative of the content area being addressed. The reader is encouraged to access the materials as primary references where desired:

- **Florida Gulf Coast University, United States. Infusing** *The Earth Charter* **into Research and Curriculum: One American University's Example** (Corcoran and Wohlpart, 2007).
- *Sustaining Life on Earth: Environmental and Human Health through Global Governance.* A multidisciplinary text containing many perspectives, each anchored in *The Earth Charter* (Soskolne et al., 2008).
- **The Use of** *The Earth Charter* **at the Primary Teacher's Education Department at the University of Crete** (Kostoulas-Makrakis, 2014).
- **Beyond Cognitive Learning: Facilitating a Reconnection between the Community and Nature at the University of Granada** (Fernández Herrería, 2014).
- **Cultivating Good Water and** *The Earth Charter.* **The Experience of Itaipu Binacional in Brazil** (Friedrich, 2014).
- *The Earth Charter* **as an Environmental Policy Instrument in Mexico: A Soft Law or Hard Policy Perspective** (Camarena Juarez, 2014).

Three of the above references (Fernández Herrería, Friedrich and Kostoulas-Makrakis) relate directly to 'Education for Sustainable Development' (ESD). These are examples of educational initiatives. One might anticipate that the number of endorsements of *The Earth Charter* would only increase with extended local initiatives. Each initiative at the local level could be anticipated to generate a groundswell of enthusiasm for the transitions that society must make if a sustainable path is to be achieved. Incentives and leadership are needed to see this movement expand.

Universal responsibility in *The Earth Charter*

The Earth Charter articulates the Principle of Universal Responsibility with extracts as follows:

> To realize these aspirations, we must decide to live with a sense of universal responsibility, identifying ourselves with the whole Earth community

as well as our local communities. We are at once citizens of different nations and of one world in which the local and global are linked.

Everyone shares responsibility for the present and future well-being of the human family and the larger living world.

The spirit of human solidarity and kinship with all life is strengthened when we live with reverence for the mystery of being, gratitude for the gift of life, and humility regarding the human place in nature.

Epidemiology and *The Earth Charter*

Epidemiology is the study of the distribution and determinants of health and disease in communities (Porta, 2014). It is a population health science. Because it examines, among other things, health effects seen in nonhuman systems with those seen in humans, it is an applied science, one that is foundational to informing rational health policy. As such, it is a complex science that must engage with other disciplines in the formulation of research hypotheses that address public health concerns. Other sciences that engage with epidemiology, or that epidemiology engages with when they consider population health questions, include, among others, biostatistics, biochemistry, biology, toxicology, industrial hygiene, sociology, anthropology, medicine, demography, but also moral philosophy and ethics.

As with other applied sciences, epidemiology rests heavily on research ethics in the formulation of hypotheses, particularly those that have implications for and require the involvement of communities. Community engagement is recognized as essential for ethical research of an epidemiological nature (International Society for Environmental Epidemiology, 2012; Kramer et al., 2012).

The ethical principles that underlie bioethics applied to human studies have strong parallels with *The Earth Charter*. Both are deontological (i.e., duty-based). The first-order principles of bioethics require the duty of respect for autonomy, beneficence, non-maleficence and distributive justice (Beauchamp and Childress, 2013). *The Earth Charter*, while not structured around the four principles as in bioethics, is a universal duty-based set of principles that extend to all life in all of its complexity.

Akin to epidemiology, *The Earth Charter* encourages interdisciplinary and transdisciplinary approaches for addressing complex social policy questions that also integrate health into all of its dimensions. In particular, *The Earth Charter* and epidemiology have 'prevention' as a focus for the support of all life and its interdependence. When environmental epidemiology, as a subspecialty of epidemiology, extends its focus to studying questions relating to the biosphere and with global implications, respecting autonomy, doing good, doing no harm and social justice permeate all such questions.

With epidemiology seeking determinants of public health, its mission is to act on these discoveries by recommending policy interventions (Porta, 2014). Since the advent of *The Earth Charter*, our attention is focussed on the most upstream of determinants. With continuing extinctions, life as we know it is declining as the global environment reaches tipping points beyond which human health itself can no longer be sustained (Ripple et al., 2017, 2020, 2021). In the absence of life-sustaining services provided by flourishing eco-systems, human health declines. It therefore falls on those in public health to focus on how the human enterprise might preserve that which supports life in all of its forms.

Prevention in this scenario, along with the application of the Precaution-ary Principle, becomes ever more paramount (Soskolne, 2005). However, through delays in action, the opportunity for prevention may well have been lost with the need now to focus more on applying the Post-Cautionary Prin-ciple (Heinzerling, 2007).

Human rights since 1948; Human duties since 2000

The Universal Declaration of Human Rights (1948) brought attention to, and fo-cussed almost exclusively on, human rights. *The Earth Charter* was introduced in 2000 as the counterbalance to human rights by identifying human duties. It became evident that, for rights to be enjoyed, duties need to be respected.

The Earth Charter is the only document that, in specifying duties:

- Supports ecological integrity rights;
- Has biocentrism at its core;
- Integrates the dependence of human health on ecological integrity and hence 'the right to life' for both present and future generations;
- Extends a right to precaution in policymaking; and
- Explicitly defends future generations.

Furthermore, *The Earth Charter* is enabling of the United Nations (UN) Sus-tainability Development Goals (SDGs) promulgated in 2015 (UN General Assembly, 2015). The SDGs (UN SDGs, 2015) provide the blueprint to bring forth a better and more sustainable future for all. They address the global challenges we face, including those related to poverty, inequality, climate, environmental degradation, prosperity and peace and justice. The Goals in-terconnect, and, in order to leave no one behind, it is important that we achieve each goal and target by 2030, consistent with the UN 2030 Agenda for Sustainable Development.

Direct connections between the SDGs and *The Earth Charter* are self-ev-ident in that both address the same global challenges. *The Earth Charter* is directly supportive of the SDGs in that it provides a set of values and ethical principles that could only aid in the attainment of the SDGs. It explicitly addresses linkages among health, poverty and conservation (as do the SDGs), and it recognizes interdependencies among all factors, particularly the up-stream determinants of health and well-being.

Addressing questions about global change through epidemiology

Under current trends, the future of life on Earth grows bleak (Ripple et al., 2017, 2020, 2021). What hope can be found in existing tools that could serve as an aid to changing our course from one of decline to one of resilience, flourishing and perhaps a path of sustainability?

With *The Earth Charter's* continual reference, explicitly and implicitly, to the upstream determinants of health and well-being, should epidemiologists bring their expertise to bear in helping the world to meet its SDGs by 2030? Would so doing make epidemiology all the more relevant in the face of global ecological change? Arguably, epidemiology has an obligation to bring its skills to help address the SDGs. Further, with *The Earth Charter's* values and ethical principles being as one with the ethics guidelines developed by the International Society for Environmental Epidemiology (ISEE, 2012; Kramer et al., 2012), the fit is a natural one to make.

As noted earlier, human health and well-being are the domain of epidemiology, which is the scientific discipline linking determinants to health/disease/well-being outcomes. Two types of determinants are recognized in the epidemiological toolkit: proximate and distal. The more upstream determinants fall into the category of distal determinants. The more distal the determinant, the more difficult it is to make connections between cause (i.e., exposure) and effect (i.e., disease) when the outcome is a rare event. However, when the outcome is not rare, making the connection is more direct.

The problem with major distal determinants, from an epidemiological perspective, is that, in the context of upstream global change determinants (e.g., climate change/global heating), once tipping points are reached and, indeed, exceeded, whole systems collapse, and the effect on people, particularly those without the buffer of wealth (and/or infrastructure), will be analogous to epidemic/pandemic phenomena. One such study showed that wealthy countries did not sustain the levels of disease and/or disintegrity of ecosystems expected; this was best explained by the buffer of wealth (Sieswerda et al., 2001). Sieswerda et al.'s (2001) study was, if not the first, among the first, epidemiological studies to demonstrate such an effect.

Because the very nature of epidemiology is to prevent harm by intervening along the causal pathway, usually through public policy, it falls on the shoulders of epidemiologists to prevent harms on a massive scale. In so doing, epidemiologists would be demonstrating solidarity, acting in the interests of both present and future generations. Such action would be in full alignment with the universal values and ethical principles comprising *The Earth Charter.*

To make the application of epidemiological methods tractable at the local level, the maxim attributed to René Dubos (1977) is relevant: 'Think globally, act locally.' This applies not only to actions needed to reduce pollution and other negative stressors arising from expanding human populations, on the biosphere, but also to epidemiologists collectively for their generation of evidence in support of rational policy for sustainability. In this way, epidemiologists, and indeed all professions, can work towards addressing matters of a global nature.

Epidemiologists concerned with the impact of global change on human health have a toolkit of methods – both quantitative and qualitative – to scientifically address questions of relevance to people around the world facing the challenge of securing a sustainable future. These methods (Ladd and Soskolne, 2008; Soskolne et al., 2008) can be applied to help inform both communities and all levels of governance about the changes needed if a sustainable path is to be achieved. The values and ethical principles of *The Earth Charter* need to be explored in relation to the endpoints identified in each of the SDGs. How linked are the SDG health-related endpoints to the values and ethics of *The Earth Charter*? The latter's values and ethics must be considered as modifiable risk factors, potential confounders and/or effect-modifiers in any epidemiological modelling.

Ethics guidelines to pave the way forward for the professions

All professions and collective action entities would likely have a mission statement and a set of core values that describe the collective motivation for the said mission. The core values also provide the anchor for each profession's activity and collective effort.

From the profession of epidemiology's subspecialty of environmental epidemiology, its Ethics Guidelines (2012) commit those considering themselves a member of such a body, to maintain, enhance and promote health in communities worldwide and to work to protect the public health interest above any other.

In moving focus away from medical or bioethics to public health ethics, environmental epidemiologists keep the four first-order principles from bioethics (i.e., respect for autonomy, beneficence, non-maleficence and distributive justice) and extend, under justice, several second- order ethical principles as follows:

- ENVIRONMENTAL JUSTICE PRINCIPLE

  Who (i.e., which community) is taking the risks?
  Who (i.e., which community) is deriving the benefits?

- POLLUTER PAYS PRINCIPLE

  Also serves as an incentive for internalizing costs.

- PRECAUTIONARY PRINCIPLE

  Requires that we act to prevent harm even if the evidence is limited.

- SEVENTH-GENERATION PRINCIPLE

  Requires that we consider the consequences of today's decisions seven generations hence.

In essence, the four first-order principles from medicine (or bioethics) are applied also in public health. In addition to these, four second-order principles are pertinent in environmental epidemiology as follows:

- Protect the most vulnerable in society (e.g., the unborn, children, indigenous populations living off the land and the frail elderly);
- Involve communities in our research to ensure the community relevance of our work;
- Integrity in public health; and
- Serve the public health interest above any other.

Equipped with these first- and second-order ethical principles, the epidemiologist should be able to address linkages along the path from upstream (distal) determinants (constituting exposures) to health, disease and well-being outcomes.

Conclusions

Humans are embedded in the ecosystems in which they live, work and play. If implemented by both individuals and collectives, with those in the wealthier countries leading globally, *The Earth Charter* would immediately shift the human enterprise from its current trajectory towards the collapse of life as we know it, to a path of sustainability.

The significance of *The Earth Charter's* values and principles were shown above in different contexts. Examples are provided of how *The Earth Charter* is being incorporated into textbooks, into governance in Mexico and from the City Government of São Paulo, Brazil, and in universities in Spain, Greece, and in Florida, USA. These examples demonstrate its utility, certainly as an educational instrument. To achieve a change in trajectory, reflections on implementing *The Earth Charter* could shed light on more effective strategies for expanding success in helping the world meet the 17 Sustainability Development Goals (SDGs) of the United Nations.

If humanity is to achieve a change in trajectory, reflections on implementing *The Earth Charter* could shed light on more effective strategies for expanding success. Near-universal adoption and endorsement of *The Earth Charter* would, however, be needed. The role of the environmental health sciences, including epidemiology, in evaluating the potential of *The Earth Charter* to limit impacts from upstream determinants of health on a scale heretofore unseen, warrants urgent consideration for the health and well-being of both present and future generations.

The role of environmental epidemiology in evaluating progress towards meeting the SDGs, and the potential of *The Earth Charter* to limit impacts from upstream determinants of health, warrants urgent consideration by humanity collectively and by the professions specifically. In particular, this chapter provides both motivation and examples for epidemiologists to consider. Attention needs to be given to adding to their research agendas, values and ethics as upstream determinants as embedded in the four domains of *The Earth Charter's* focus (i.e., Respect and Care for the Community of Life; Ecological Integrity; Social and Economic Justice; and Democracy, Nonviolence and Peace).

Consistent with their own ethics guidelines, community engagement with epidemiologists is warranted as they move their research agendas forward to include questions relating to the upstream determinants of global sustainability. Evidence so generated could provide the rational basis for policy shifts to a path of sustainability, from the local to the global, and vice versa.

Acknowledgement

Mirian Vilela, Executive Director, Earth Charter International, University for Peace, Costa Rica, kindly assisted in providing reference to five of the six case studies in advance of the presentation in 2018 upon which this chapter is based.

References

Arrhenius S. (1896). On the influence of carbonic acid in the air upon the temperature of the ground. *The London, Edinburgh, and Dublin Philosophical Magazine and Journal of Science*. 41 (251): 237–276. doi:10.1080/14786449608620846 (accessed 12 September 2021).
Beauchamp TL and Childress JF. (2013). *Principles of Biomedical Ethics* (7th Ed.). Oxford University Press, New York.
Butler CD. (2016). Sounding the alarm: Health in the Anthropocene. *International Journal of Environmental Research and Public Health*. 13 (7): 665 (15 pages). Published online 2016 Jun 30. https://www.mdpi.com/1660-4601/13/7/665 (accessed 12 September 2021).
Camarena Juarez FJ. (2014). *The Earth Charter* as an environmental policy instrument in Mexico: A soft law or hard policy perspective (2014). Chapter 19. In: Westra L and Vilela M (Editors) *The Earth Charter, Ecological Integrity and Social Movements*. Earthscan from Routledge, Taylor & Francis, London and New York. pp. 230–243.
Corcoran PB and Wohlpart AJ. (2007). Infusing the Earth Charter into research and curriculum: One American University's example. In: *Good Practices in Education for Sustainable Development Using the Earth Charter: UNESCO/ Earth Charter International. Education for Sustainable Development in Action*. pp. 110–114. Entire document can be downloaded at https://earthcharter.org/library/good-practices-using-the-earth-charter-2/ (accessed 12 September 2021).
Cranor CF. (2011). *Legally Poisoned: How the Law Puts Us at Risk from Toxicants*. Harvard University Press, Cambridge, MA.

Dubos R. (1977). René Dubos. From Wikipedia, the free encyclopedia. https://en.wikipedia.org/wiki/Ren%C3%A9_Dubos (accessed 12 September 2021).

Ehrlich PR and Holdren JP. (1971). Impact of population growth. *Science*. 171 (3977): 1212–1217. doi: 10.1126/science.171.3977.1212 (accessed 12 September 2021).

Fernández Herrería A. (2014). Beyond cognitive learning: Facilitating a reconnection between the community and nature at the University of Granada. In: *The Heart of the Matter: Infusing Sustainability Values in Education: Experiences of ESD with the Earth Charter* (publicación digitalizada)/editado por Alicia Jiménez Elizondo y Douglas F. Williamson. – San José, C.R.: Universidad para la Paz. pp. 79–83. Entire book can be downloaded at https://www.academia.edu/9972981/The_Heart_of_the_Matter_Infusing_Sustainability_Values_in_Education (accessed 12 September 2021).

Friedrich N. (2014). Cultivating good water and *The Earth Charter*. The experience of Itaipu Binacional in Brazil. In: *The Heart of the Matter: Infusing Sustainability Values in Education: Experiences of ESD with the Earth Charter* (publicación digitalizada)/editado por Alicia Jiménez Elizondo y Douglas F. Williamson. – San José, C.R.: Universidad para la Paz. pp. 20–24. Entire book can be downloaded at https://www.academia.edu/9972981/The_Heart_of_the_Matter_Infusing_Sustainability_Values_in_Education (accessed 12 September 2021).

Heinzerling L. (2007). Climate Change, Human Health, and the Post-Cautionary Principle. *Georgetown University Law Center*. http://ssrn.com/AbstractID=1008923 (accessed 12 September 2021).

International Society for Environmental Epidemiology (ISEE). (2012). Ethics Guidelines for Environmental Epidemiologists, April 25, 2012. https://www.iseepi.org/docs/ISEE_Ethics_Guidelines_adopted_april_25_2012-English.pdf (accessed 12 September 2021).

Kostoulas-Makrakis N. (2014). The use of the Earth Charter at the Primary Teachers Education Department, University of Crete, Greece. In: *The Heart of the Matter: Infusing Sustainability Values in Education: Experiences of ESD with The Earth Charter*. (publicación digitalizada)/editado por Alicia Jiménez Elizondo y Douglas F. Williamson. – San José, C.R.: Universidad para la Paz. pp. 91–95. Entire book can be downloaded at https://www.academia.edu/9972981/The_Heart_of_the_Matter_Infusing_Sustainability_Values_in_Education (accessed 12 September 2021).

Kramer S, Soskolne CL, Mustapha BA and Al-Delaimy WK. (2012). Revised ethics guidelines for environmental epidemiologists. (Editorial.) *Environmental Health Perspectives*. 120 (8): A299–A301. http://www.ncbi.nlm.nih.gov/pmc/articles/PMC3440101/pdf/ehp.1205562.pdf (accessed 12 September 2021).

Ladd BD and Soskolne CL. (2008). A toolkit for ecoepidemiological enquiry under global ecological change. In: Soskolne CL, Westra L, Kotzé LJ, Mackey B, Rees WE and Westra R (Editors) *Sustaining Life on Earth: Environmental and Human Health through Global Governance*. Lexington Books, a Division of Rowman & Littlefield Publishers, Inc., Lanham, MD (482 pages). pp. 369–382.

McMichael AJ. (1993). *Planetary Overload: Global Environmental Change and the Health of the Human Species*. Cambridge University Press, Cambridge.

Meadows DH, Meadows DL, Randers J and Behrens III WW. (1972). *The Limits to Growth: A Report for the Club of Rome's Project on the Predicament of Mankind*. Universe Books, New York. http://www.donellameadows.org/wp-content/userfiles/Limits-to-Growth-digital-scan-version.pdf (accessed 12 September 2021).

Porta M. (Editor) (2014). *A Dictionary of Epidemiology* (6th Ed.). Oxford University Press, New York.

Ripple WJ, Wolf C, Newsome TM, Galetti M, Alamgir M, Crist E, Mahmoud MI and Laurance WF. (2017). World scientists' warning to humanity: A second notice. *BioScience.* 67 (12): 1026–1028. https://doi.org/10.1093/biosci/bix125 (accessed 12 September 2021).

Ripple WJ, Wolf C, Newsome TM, Barnard P, Moomaw WR. (2020). World scientists' warning of a climate emergency. *BioScience.* 70 (1): 8–12. https://doi.org/10.1093/biosci/biz088 (accessed 12 September 2021).

Ripple WJ, Wolf C, Newsome TM, Gregg JW, Lenton TM, Palomo I, Eikel-boom JAJ, Law BE, Huq S, Duffy PB and Rockström J. (2021). World Scientists' Warning of a Climate Emergency 2021. *BioScience.* 71 (9): 894–898. https://doi.org/10.1093/biosci/biab079 (accessed 12 September 2021).

Sieswerda LE, Soskolne CL, Newman SC, Schopflocher D and Smoyer KE. (2001). Toward measuring the impact of ecological disintegrity on human health. *Epidemiology.* 12 (1): 28–32. https://www.jstor.org/stable/3703675?seq=1#page_scan_tab_contents (accessed 12 September 2021).

Soskolne CL and Bertollini R. (1999). Global ecological integrity and 'sustainable development': Cornerstones of public health. A Discussion Document. http://www.colinsoskolne.com/documents/WHO-1999_Discussion_Document.pdf (accessed 12 September 2021).

Soskolne CL. (2003). Measuring the impact of ecological disintegrity on human health: A role for epidemiology. Chapter 29 In: Rapport DJ, WL Lasley, DE Rolston, NO Nielsen, CO Qualset and AB Damania (Editors) *Managing for Healthy Ecosystems.* Lewis Publishers, Boca Raton, FL. ISBN: 1566706122 (1,510 pages). pp. 259–265.

Soskolne CL. (2005). On the even greater need for precaution under global change (Reprinted from The European Journal of Oncology Library, Vol 2, 2003). *Human and Ecological Risk Assessment.* 11(1): 97–106.

Soskolne CL, Huynen M, Ladd BD and Martens P. (2008). Eco-epidemiological enquiry under global ecological change: An integrated assessment toolkit for beginners. *European Journal of Oncology.* Ramazzini Library. http://www.collegiumramazzini.org/gest/up/Sosklone.pdf; http://www.collegiumramazzini.org/download/SOSKOLNE07.pdf (accessed 12 September 2021).

Soskolne CL, Westra L, Kotzé LJ, Mackey B, Rees WE and Westra R (Editors) (2008). *Sustaining Life on Earth: Environmental and Human Health through Global Governance.* Lexington Books, a Division of Rowman & Littlefield Publishers, Inc., Lanham, MD. p. 482. http://www.LexingtonBooks.com/ISBN/0739117297 (accessed 12 September 2021).

Soskolne CL. (2017). Global, regional and local ecological change: Ethical, aspects of public health research and practice. Chapter 1 In: Zölzer F and Meskens G (Editors) *Ethics of Environmental Health. Routledge Studies in Environment and Health.* Routledge, Taylor & Francis. London and New York. pp. 3–16.

Soskolne CL. (2019). The role of vested interests and dominant narratives in science, risk management and risk communication. Chapter 8 In: Zölzer F and Meskens G (Editors) *Environmental Health Risks: Ethical Aspects. Routledge Studies in Environment and Health.* Routledge, Taylor & Francis, London and New York. pp. 123–134.

The Earth Charter. (2000). http://earthcharter.org/discover/download-the-charter/ (accessed 12 September 2021).

The Earth Charter. (2019). https://en.wikipedia.org/wiki/Earth_Charter. For endorsements, see 'Reaction …' (accessed 12 September 2021).

UN General Assembly. (2015). Transforming our world: The 2030 agenda for sustainable development. 21 October 2015, A/RES/70/1. https://www.refworld.org/docid/57b6e3e44.html (accessed 12 September 2021).

UN Sustainability Development Goals (SDGs). (2015). http://www.un.org/sustainabledevelopment/sustainable-development-goals/ (accessed 12 September 2021).

Universal Declaration of Human Rights. (1948). United Nations General Assembly, Paris. 10 December 1948 (General Assembly resolution 217 A). https://www.un.org/en/universal-declaration-human-rights/ (accessed 12 September 2021).

3 Cosmopolitanism and environmental health

Gaston Meskens

Intro cosmopolitanism and environmental health

The concept of 'environmental health' knows multiple understandings. In a scientific spirit, it may be characterised as '... *the branch of public health concerned with all aspects of the natural and built environment affecting human health ...*' with the major sub-disciplines being '... *environmental science, environmental and occupational medicine, toxicology and epidemiology...*' (Wikipedia 2020). From a normative perspective on environmental health risk governance, it can be described as '... *involving the assessment and control of environmental factors that can potentially affect human health, such as radiation, toxic chemicals and other hazardous agents ...*', bearing in mind that '... *ethical frameworks and underpinnings that guide environmental health research and regulation are not always made explicit and [...] require greater attention ...*' (Zölzer and Meskens 2017, 2019).

While these descriptions suggest specific pragmatic or ethical approaches focussing on 'the problem and the cure', the concept of environmental health can also be understood in a more 'spiritual' holistic way as striving for the collective of human beings to live in harmony (instead of in tension) with their natural habitat. This understanding has already inspired and influenced actual visions on environmental health governance. Two important examples of global governance may illustrate this. Back in 2009, the United Nations General Assembly (UNGA) adopted its first resolution on 'Harmony with Nature'. The idea was that '... *the Earth and its ecosystems are our common home ...*' and so the UNGA member-states '... *expressed their conviction that it is necessary to promote Harmony with Nature in order to achieve a just balance among the economic, social and environmental needs of present and future generations ...*' (United Nations n.d.; UNGA 2009). As a second example, it is worth mentioning the Earth Charter. This charter came into being in 1994 on initiative of Maurice Strong (the then Secretary-General of the Rio Earth Summit) and Mikhail Gorbachev (former President of the Soviet Union) through the organisations they each founded (the Earth Council and the Green Cross International respectively). The first article of the Charter sets the tone for a clearly holistic vision on life on earth, stating that one should '... *Respect Earth and life in all its diversity ...*' and '... *Recognize that all*

DOI: 10.4324/9780429318436-5

beings are interdependent and every form of life has value regardless of its worth to human beings…' (The Earth Charter n.d. Article 1).

This chapter takes another specific approach to making sense of environmental health, although with the aim to situate it into the holistic understanding of environmental health referred to above. Obviously attention will be given to the 'problem and cure' approach to environmental health as specified in the two first citations, but the main argument of the first section of this chapter will be why – in the interest of fair and effective environmental health governance – we need to initially focus on the character of complexity of our environmental health problems and on what it would imply to deal with them in a fair way. Today, environmental health problems are complex problems, and the argument will be that a fair dealing with these problems implies a fair dealing with their complexity and that our joint responsible attitude when making sense of the complexity of those problems can be described as a 'reflexive attitude in face of that complexity'. In conclusion, the chapter will propose a specific 'ethics of care' vision on how to deal with environmental health problems, given that we are all 'bound in complexity' facing those problems.

When the ancient Greeks started to speak of 'cosmopolitanism' in the 4th century BC, the world was still a fairly simple place to live as compared to today. Their interpretation of what it meant to be 'a citizen of the world' was well intended but merely 'spiritual' and not so much influenced by the 'reality' of that world. Today, the situation is dramatically different. The fact of globalisation and of the interconnectedness of our current socioeconomic practices, together with the given that complex environmental health problems now manifest worldwide and on global scale, instructs a global perspective for both interpretation of and approach to these problems. Today, we have to understand that, as individuals enjoying an acceptable standard of living in our contemporary society, all of our choices with respect to the food we eat, the clothes we wear, the consumer products we buy, the energy we consume, the means of transport we use and so on have some effect on either a global scale or at least an effect somewhere else on earth. Humanity is now a globally connected collective of human beings who all influence and depend on each other. As a consequence, moral reasoning with respect to those choices requires us to look beyond our familiar local 'comfort zones' and to think as 'citizens of the world' or 'cosmopolitans' who try to evaluate the consequences of their choices and who are motivated to understand their specific place, role, responsibilities and rights in the (global) bigger picture of it all. From that perspective, section 2 concludes with the thought that, whether in the interest of environmental health or of other complex social problems, dealing fairly with each other in that connected collective implies a fair dealing with the global complexity of influences and dependences that binds us. Therefore, cosmopolitanism, as an ancient ethical concept, is not any longer a spiritual abstract idea but a fundamental normative vision on humanity and the world we cannot deny.

Based on these introductory sections, the chapter then elaborates on a connection between the current need 'to deal fairly' with the complexity that binds us on the one hand and the need to think and act as cosmopolitans on the other. Building on the 'ethics of care' vision 'in face of complexity' proposed in the first section, and on the observation from the second section that cosmopolitan thinking is no longer a choice but a necessity, the third and fourth sections will propose a specific contemporary meaning of cosmopolitanism, its motivations and its character as a moral stance and will conclude with a reflection on the meaning of 'cosmopolitanism as ethical competence' and how it is a fundamental requirement for sustainable and fair environmental health governance.

On the 13th of January 2020, the World Health Organization released a statement entitled 'Urgent Health Challenges for the Next Decade'. In that statement, the WHO noted that

> We need to realize that health is an investment in the future. Countries invest heavily in protecting their people from terrorist attacks, but not against the attack of a virus, which could be far more deadly, and far more damaging economically and socially. A pandemic could bring economies and nations to their knees. Which is why health security cannot be a matter for ministries of health alone.
>
> (World Health Organization 2020)

Whether or not the authors were already foreseeing the 2020 pandemic caused by the outbreak and the worldwide spread of the SARS-CoV-2-virus, for sure we can say we now live in a different world as compared to when their words were published in January 2020. The challenges coming with controlling and preventing a health crisis of this character and scale may be seen as an extra motivation to understand and deliberate upon environmental health governance from a holistic and cosmopolitan ethics of care perspective.

The fact of complexity of environmental health governance

What comprises environmental health? In the preamble to its constitution, the WHO states that '… *Health is a state of complete physical, mental and social well-being and not merely the absence of disease or infirmity….*' (World Health Organization n.d.). In combination with the general description of environmental health quoted above, being '*the branch of public health concerned with all aspects of the natural and built environment affecting human health*', one could possibly understand environmental health as being 'only' concerned with those 'tangible' aspects of the natural and built environment affecting physical, mental and social well-being and not with, for example, social, economic or political aspects. However, given that the references above further specify that subdisciplines of environmental health (as a public research and policy practice) are environmental science, environmental and occupational medicine, toxicology and epidemiology and that the focus is on 'hazardous agents' such as toxic chemicals and radiation, we can conclude that we should understand the natural and built environment as 'affected' or 'distorted' environments and not as pure or idealistic environments. Furthermore, it is clear we should understand these environments as being affected or distorted by human activity and that this human activity can manifest in complex, indirect and often invisible ways. To give just two examples: massive populations of insects and earthquakes are both 'aspects of the natural environment', but human activity may certainly have influence on their cause and effect. Evidence is supporting the hypothesis that there is a link between the 2020 locusts plague in East Africa and climate change resulting in ocean temperature gradient disturbance and consequent extreme wet weather (Stone 2020). Earthquakes – although in lighter form – are now observed as being caused by natural gas field exploitation, while 'natural' earthquakes have greater adverse effects on people living in poor urban conditions. These two examples may already show the complexity of grasping environmental health phenomena, but this is not the end of the story, as causality should not only be understood in a natural or technical way but also as comprising economic, social, political and even spiritual factors. The seed politics of transnational corporations such as Monsanto-Bayer supported by (or rather 'not hindered by') national and international regulation is a deplorable example of how economic and political factors can have direct adverse effects on local farmers' health and well-being (see, among others, Busscher et al. 2020; Peschard and Randeria 2020). The emergence of megacities is an example of how socioeconomic factors influencing the built environment can have adverse consequences on physical, mental and social well-being of citizens (among others, see Liu et al. 2016; Rodwin and Gusmano 2002). And, obviously, climate change might be the best example of how socioeconomic and related political factors now disturb the natural environment to a scale never seen before.

With health being defined by the WHO as 'the state of complete physical, mental and social well-being', the examples above may show that 'environmental health' focussing on 'aspects of the natural and built environment' is nothing more than a specific lens to look at the broad and complex field of health governance in general and at specific cases in particular. That lens is however an interesting one, for it provides a meaningful 'practical' way to situate environmental health issues in the bigger picture and to understand them as problems complicated by natural, technical, social, economic and political factors. Today, environmental health problems are complex problems, in the first place because they are troubled by knowledge-related uncertainties and diverse and often incommensurable value-based interpretations. Second, complexity can also be due to the interconnectedness of problems (which means that they cannot be tackled separately) or their diversified impacts in character and time. As a consequence, our responsibilities with respect to these problems are diversified and 'relative' in relation to others' responsibilities. Because of all this, all complex environmental health problems listed above are first and foremost complex *social* problems, instead of only scientific, technical or environmental problems.

In Meskens (2017), I proposed to understand complex social problems as all having the same seven characteristics, and I propose here that also complex environmental health problems, as a 'subset' of complex social problems, can be characterised in this way:

A NEUTRAL CHARACTERIZATION OF COMPLEXITY: SEVEN CHARACTERISTICS OF COMPLEX ENVIRON-MENTAL HEALTH PROBLEMS (MESKENS 2017)

1   Diversified impact
- Individuals and/or groups are affected by the problem in diverse ways (benefit vs. adverse consequence, diverse 'degrees' of benefits or adverse consequences).
- The impact can be economic or related to physical or psychic health, or individual or collective social well-being.
- The character and degree of impact may evolve or vary in a contingent way in time.
- The impact may also manifest later in time (with the possibility that it manifests after or during several generations).

2   Interdependence
- The problem is caused and/or influenced by multiple factors (social, economic, technical, natural) and relates itself to other problems.
- Interdependence can change in time.
- The context of concern becomes global.

3   The need for a 'broader' coherent approach (organisational complexity)
    Due to diversified impact and interdependence, problems need to be tackled 'together' in a coherent, systematic and 'holistic' approach. This approach needs to take into account the following four additional characteristics of complexity:

4   Relative responsibilities
    Due to diversified impact, interdependence and organisational complexity, responsibility cannot be assigned to one specific actor. Responsibilities are relative in two ways:
- (1) Mutual: the possibility for one actor to take responsibility can depend on whether another actor takes responsibility or not;
- (2) Collective: our collective responsibility is relative in the sense that it will need to be 'handed over' to a next 'collective' (a new government, next generations).

5 Knowledge-related uncertainty (knowledge problem)
   Analysis of the problem is complicated by uncertainty due to speculative, incomplete or contradictory knowledge, with respect to the character and evolution of impact and interdependence and with respect to the effects of the coherent and holistic approach.

6 Value pluralism (evaluation problem)
   Evaluation of diversified impact, interdependence and organisational complexity and of subsequent relative responsibilities is complicated due to

   – the knowledge problem;
   – the existence of different visions based on different specific values and world views;
   – the existence of different interests of concerned actors;
   – the fact that it is therefore impossible to determine in consensus what would be the 'real' problem or the 'root' of the problem;
   – the fact that 'meta-values' such as 'equality', 'freedom' and 'sustainability' cannot be translated unambiguously into practical responsibilities or actions.

7 Relative authorities (authority problem)
   The authority of actors who evaluate and judge the problem and rationalise their interests and responsibilities related to it in a future-oriented perspective is relative in two ways:

   – The 'individual' authority of concerned actors is relative in the sense that, due to the knowledge and evaluation problem, authority cannot be 'demonstrated' or 'enforced' purely on the basis of knowledge or judgement. As a consequence, that authority needs to lean on 'external' references (the mandate of the elected politician, the diplomas and experience of the scientific expert, the commercial success of the entrepreneur, the social status of the spiritual leader, the appeal to justice of the activist etc.).
   – The 'collective' authority of concerned actors who operate within the traditional governing modes of politics, science and the market is relative, as these governing modes cannot rely on an objective 'authority of method': the systems of representative democracy (through party politics and elections) and the market both lean on the principle of competition, while science is faced with the fact that it needs to deal with future-oriented hypotheses.

   As such, concerned actors have the opportunity to reject or question the relevance and credibility of the judgement of other actors and, consequently, to question the legitimacy of their authority.

It may be clear from the descriptions that characteristics 1, 2 and 3 could be called characteristics of a 'factual complexity' and that 5, 6 and 7 refer to a complexity of interpretation as a consequence of that factual complexity. Number 4 (relative responsibilities) might be described as a 'combination' of a factual complexity and a complexity of interpretation: the fact that a concerned actor does (not) act according to their responsibility may have practical consequences for other actors, also in terms of their own ability to act responsibly. On the other hand, the actor's motivation to act according to their responsibility is of course also dependent on their interpretation of the situation and of arguments of others with respect to their responsibility.

Due to their factual complexity, complex environmental health problems are problems that 'create themselves' uncertainty and ambiguity related to what is at stake and what is to be done. The complexity of interpretation may thus be understood as a complexity of making sense of the problem. As this complexity also includes 'the authority problem', the complexity of interpretation of a complex environmental health problem can be understood as a complexity that is, in principle, experienced by all concerned actors 'together' and not only by each actor individually.

I will elaborate further on the consequences of this 'fact of complexity' of complex environmental health problems in section 3. For now, while we recognise the similar character of complexity of complex environmental health problems, it is also important to focus on their meaningful differences. Complex environmental health problems have one or more specific health risks as their central concern, and, from that perspective, it is also important to distinguish them on the basis of our ability to deal with those health risks as potentially affected on the one hand and on the basis of our ability as society to possibly justify or avoid the situations and practices at the origin of these risks on the other. Living conditions such as living in slums or poverty in general are known threats to health and can never be justified as such. A non–communicable disease such as cancer can be seen as 'simply belonging to the natural cycle of life and death', which doesn't mean that we cannot try to avoid or treat it. As humans always risking cancer, our behaviour is crucial for our health, but so is our ability to reason about the risk coming with it and the access to information and treatment. The same can be said about communicable diseases such as flu, HIV and the recently emerged Covid-19, although the fact that these diseases are communicable obviously puts an extra responsibility on us, as our behaviour can not only put our own health in danger but also that of those around us, including those we specially care about. In terms of how we can possibly deal with environmental health risks, a special (and large) category are those that come with practices that concern society at large and of which the associated health risks might as such be justified as 'acceptable' under certain circumstances. Typical examples of these practices are the food and pharmacy industry, industrial farming, mining, the use of potentially hazardous consumer products or mobile phones and the use of nuclear energy or fossil fuels. It may be clear that the common denominator of these practices is their reliance on science and technology. For these 'industrial and technological (health) risks', the traditional understanding is that a specific 'level' of risk can be considered acceptable in view of the benefits the practice would bring, and our ability to deal with these practices and risks as potentially affected depends on whether we have a say in justifying them as well as on our ability to protect ourselves against the risk.

In general, we could say that our ability to deal with environmental health risks will depend on practical possibilities instructed by specific rights and values. In that sense, the right to information about the risk, the right to protection and care, and the value of precaution are commonly meaningful and essential for dealing with diseases, unacceptable living conditions and industrial and technological risks. For what the justification of industrial and technological risks is concerned, also the right to co-decide and the value of informed consent can be called meaningful and essential.[1] For communicable and non-communicable diseases, it is clear that under no conditions people would voluntarily consent to a disease, although given that now everyone is aware of the risk of smoking, smokers could be said to give informed consent to the possibility of lung cancer. In medical context, the value of informed consent is important as such, as it becomes meaningful and essential in the context of diagnosis and treatment of diseases. Last but not least, the right to co-decide and the value of informed consent can be called meaningful and essential in governance of protection measures for communicable diseases that could affect the wider population (such as Covid-19).

What do we learn from this short reflection on 'the fact of complexity' of environmental health problems? First, grasping complex environmental health problems requires to see them in 'the bigger picture', taking into account not only 'aspects of the natural and built environment' but also and, foremost, the social, economic and political factors influencing ('affecting') these environments. Second, thinking about our ability to deal with these problems, either as potentially affected individuals or as a society trying to grasp and govern these problems, the 'fact' of the influence of these social, economic and political factors urges us to see the potentially affected not only as passive undergoers but also and foremost as active citizens having a role in dealing effectively and fairly with these problems. If fairness is understood as 'impartial and just treatment or behaviour without favouritism or discrimination' then the role of citizens can be understood as twofold and instructed by their rights as well as responsibilities. The right to co-decide on environmental health issues that might potentially affect us as citizens is inseparable from the need to take our own responsibility with regard to these issues, although the second requires the first as condition. In other words, the motivation and ability of the potentially affected to take their responsibility can only be grounded in their ability to make sense of the issue and of their own and others' responsible behaviour in relation to it. Those others are not only our fellow citizens but also and especially the political mandatories and the various social and economic power holders who initiate and manage practices and situations (potentially) causing environmental health risks. The ethics of environmental health should therefore refer not only to our own responsible behaviour or to 'good governance' manifested in the form of socio-technical safety measures and/or environmental regulation but also and foremost to values inspiring an ethical approach to the socio-politics of environmental health governance, such as informed consent, transdisciplinarity, participation of the potentially affected, and capacity building for participation.

This last argument will be further elaborated in section 4. What is important at this stage of the reasoning is a reflection on the global character of complex environmental health problems. Not only may environmental health problems have local causes and global impact (such as climate change or the Covid-19 pandemic) or a 'global cause' with local impacts (such as the globalised economy resulting in local deforestation and land degradation); their interdependence (the second characteristic of their complexity), too, unavoidably, stretches the context of concern to the global level. Knowing that caring about (and thinking through) the global perspective is what can be called 'cosmopolitanism', a reflection on the possible meaning of this concept for the better of environmental health governance will be the subject of the next section.

The fate and rescue of cosmopolitanism

Similar to the concept of environmental health, cosmopolitanism today knows multiple meanings. The origin of the idea is to be situated in the ancient Greek culture of the Cynics during the 4th century BC. A 'cosmopolitan' was a 'citizen of the cosmos' and, as emphasized by the author Kwame Anthony Appiah, that expression was meant to be paradoxical, reflecting the general Cynic scepticism toward custom and tradition:

> A citizen – a polítēs – belonged to a particular polis, a city to which he or she owed loyalty. The cosmos referred to the world, not in the sense of the earth, but in the sense of the universe. Talk of cosmopolitanism originally signalled, then, a rejection of the conventional view that every civilized person belonged to a community among communities.
>
> (Appiah 2015)

The Greek thereafter inspired the Romans, and especially the Roman Stoics. According to Appiah, particularly the Roman Emperor Marcus Aurelius expressed himself as a 'cosmopolitan' in his writings (now known as the *Meditations*), leaning on the 'cosmopolitan conviction of the oneness of humanity' (Appiah 2015, xii). As the philosopher Anthony Clifford Grayling writes,

> In the Meditations, Marcus Aurelius expresses the view that the universe is an organic living whole, in which everything is related to everything else, and in which human individuals are 'limbs' of the whole. It follows

that the well-being of individuals is dependent upon the well-being of everything else. In the same way, each individual is inseparably an organic part of his society, so that individual good cannot be detached from the good of the collective.

(Marcus Aurelius 2002, preface by A.C. Grayling)

A reflection on how the idea of cosmopolitanism subsequently lived (or not) throughout 'Western' history (the Middle Ages, the Renaissance, the Enlightenment, Modernity) or in other civilisations is beyond the scope of this chapter. A general thought however is that these ideas, in whatever form of context, were merely 'spiritual', in the sense of 'not influenced by reality', given that conceptions and real-life experiences of the world as a physical globe on the one hand and of other cultures on the other hand only started to manifest when sailors embarked to explore the seas. A history of the idea of cosmopolitanism, however, is not needed in the context of this chapter. What matters here is the difference between what was then and what is now, and that difference is important. Since the first conception by the Greeks until modern times, the old cosmopolitan ideas that 'we are all in this together' and that we have obligations towards others (i.e., others broader than the close circle around us) may have had a variety of conceptual meanings, but never a practical urge. In that sense, if Marcus Aurelius was convinced that 'the well-being of individuals is dependent upon the well-being of everything else', we may understand his view may be called normative-spiritual but not necessarily instructed by reality. In the 'community among communities', one could bother about how to position oneself towards the communities next door, but there were certainly no problems of a wider, let stand global, scale to collectively deal with. Sure the Greek and the Romans were travellers, and so were Vasco da Gama, Christopher Columbus, Ferdinand Magellan and, later, Stanley and Livingstone. But their expeditions were meant to explore, exploit and conquer rather than to seek rapprochement with the aim to deliberate problems of a wider scale.

Today, the situation is dramatically different. The fact of globalisation and of the interconnectedness of our current socioeconomic practices,[2] together with the given that complex environmental health problems now manifest worldwide and on global scale, instructs not only a holistic but also a global perspective for both the interpretation of and the approach to these problems. Climate change may again be the best example to illustrate this, but the food industry, too, brings along concerns related to environmental health that are now of global scale. In addition, it is known that the problem of climate change is closely interconnected with the problems of the food industry in multiple ways. The reason is that environmental health risks created by the food industry include not only 'direct' and 'local' risks to our health, such as with the use of pesticides, but also indirect risks that manifest globally and in the longer term, such as loss of biodiversity and land degradation.[3] The best example of interconnectedness of global environmental health problems may now be the way the Covid-19 pandemic that broke out in 2020 is said to be linked with 'the rampant destruction of the natural world' (Carrington 2020). If, for many citizens of the world, globalisation and interconnectedness were still abstract phenomena before, the way Covid-19 impacted the world since 2020 make these phenomena directly tangible in the daily lives of all of us.

Taking all this into account, it may be clear that environmental health governance would benefit from a global perspective for both interpretation and approach. Typically, the examples of climate change, unsustainable food production and consumption, and the Covid-19 pandemic illustrate thereby that not only politicians, experts or entrepreneurs have the responsibility to apply this global perspective as a measure to evaluate their own visions and acts, but actually all of us, as citizens, are bound to that responsibility when we make choices that have an impact on environmental health (such as the choice to eat meat, or not). Today, we have to understand that, as individuals enjoying an acceptable standard of living in our contemporary society, all of our choices with respect to the food we eat, the clothes we wear, the consumer products we buy, the energy we consume, the means of transport we use and so on have some effect on a global scale or at least somewhere else on earth. We are all 'connected in complexity', and, as a consequence, ethical reasoning with respect to those choices requires us to look beyond our familiar local 'comfort zones' and to think as 'citizens of the world' or cosmopolitans who try to evaluate the consequences of their choices and who are motivated to understand their specific place, role, rights and responsibilities in the bigger picture of it all.

Obviously, this view raises questions about what this all means considering the different conditions and settings people live in. On the one hand, it is reasonable to say it is not only the responsibility of those enjoying an acceptable standard of living to think and act as cosmopolitans. On the other hand, we understand that those trying to survive in a slum couldn't care less about whether they are cosmopolitans and what that would mean. This issue will be taken up again in section 4. For now, the main conclusion here is that, today, *we have no choice but to perceive the concept of cosmopolitanism from out of the context of our social reality.* In his Meditations, Marcus Aurelius wrote at some point:

> In one way humanity touches me very nearly, inasmuch as I am bound to do good to my fellow creatures and bear with them. On the other hand, to the extent that individual men hamper my proper activities, humanity becomes a thing as indifferent to me as the sun, the wind, or the creatures of the wild. True, others may hinder the carrying out of certain actions; but they cannot obstruct my will, nor the disposition of my mind, since these will always safeguard themselves under reservations and adapt themselves to circumstances.
>
> (Marcus Aurelius 2002, Book V, note 20)

We know Marcus Aurelius was not only a pacifist and a philosopher who promoted the value of cosmopolitanism, but also an emperor who had a hard time dealing with famine, pestilences and aggressive intruders at the borders of the immense empire he inherited from his predecessors. The quote should thus not be understood as a relativisation of his own cosmopolitan stance but rather as a way to refer to the belief in what he thought was needed to do. Evidently, there is nothing wrong with such a belief. Today, however, indifference towards humanity is no longer an option. Humanity is now a globally connected collective of human beings who all influence and depend on each other. Whether in the interest of environmental health or of other complex social problems, dealing fairly with each other in that connected collective implies a fair dealing with the complexity of influences and dependences that binds us. And this requires us to be reflexive about our beliefs, interests, hopes, hypotheses and concerns related to these influences and dependences and to evaluate them in the bigger cosmopolitan picture of it all.[4] Cosmopolitanism, as an ancient ethical concept, is rescued today from detached spiritual musings and imposed on us as a fundamental vision on humanity and the world, not because we all want it, but because we have no choice.

Cosmopolitanism as an ethics of reflexivity, 'bound in complexity'

What do we learn from the previous reasoning with regard to the understanding of cosmopolitanism, in particular in relation to our individual behaviour? The first thing is that, for all of us, striving for that 'acceptable standard of living' (a house, a car, a mobile phone, in addition to access to affordable and decent goods and services provided by the market and/or the government) can no longer be done from out of something 'smaller' than a cosmopolitan perspective. As a collective global human society, not only many of our choices and acts have global consequences, we also rely on global systems, dynamics and evolutions for important aspects of our lives. Today, thinking and acting as a cosmopolitan is therefore not a moral choice you can make yourself. You might try to live 'responsibly disconnected', with your own grown food, natural medicine and a hut in the woods, but every additional – even eco-friendly – 'luxury' (a bike, solar panels, etc.) makes you immediately dependent on a global market. In addition, today digital literacy and a digital connection to the world are no longer an option but a condition to function as a citizen in a society that relies more and more on services provided through the web. The consequence is that a phone and/ or a computer became a bare necessity next to food, water and shelter, although one that is provided by a global market that heavily depends on cheap labour and even slavery.[5] Second, today, the moral appeal to 'think and act cosmopolitan' sounds everywhere around us, if only because the media and the Internet now provide 'windows on the world' in constant streams. Sure we can choose to deny that appeal and not bother about the fate of others and nature, but the fact that we live in that 'globally connected collective' makes us to understand not only that claiming our freedom of behaviour may directly harm others but also that the harmful consequences of our own and others' behaviour will always come back to us in one way or another. In other words, the character of complexity of environmental health problems makes that we are all 'bound' in that complexity. In Meskens (2017), I argued that the 'fact of complexity' brings along three new characteristics of modern coexistence that can be named 'connectedness', 'vulnerability' and 'sense of engagement'. Their meaning in relation to the complexity of complex social problems in general and of environmental health problems in particular can be summarised as follows:

Connectedness

We are connected with each other 'in complexity'. We cannot any longer escape or avoid it. Fair dealing with each other implies fair dealing with the complexity that binds us.

Vulnerability

In complexity, we became intellectually dependent on each other while we face our own and each other's 'authority problem'. We should care for the vulnerability of the ignorant and the confused, but also for that of 'mandated authority' (such as that of the scientific expert, the politician or the teacher). Last but not least, we should care for the vulnerability of those who cannot be involved in joint reflection and deliberation at all. Obviously, without wanting to make evaluative comparisons between them, these can be identified as the next generations but also as those among us who are intellectually incapable of joining (children, those who may be unconscious or otherwise incapacitated, or with serious mental disabilities).

(Sense of) Engagement

As modern human beings, our experiences now extend from the local to the global. As intelligent reflective beings, becoming involved in deliberating issues of general societal concern became a new source of meaning and moral motivation for each one of us. As citizens, we want to enjoy the right to be responsible in the complexity that binds us, although not only in our own interest. The idea is that, for contemporary humans, the will to contribute to making sense of the complexity of our coexistence in general, and of the complexity of issues such as environmental health governance in particular, can be understood as driven by an *intellectual need* and as *a form of 'intellectual' altruism*. The contemporary human becomes frustrated and unhappy if she/he is unable to put that social engagement into practice in one way or another.[6]

The focus of this chapter does not allow deeper elaboration on the meaning-fulness of these characteristics or on how they would manifest in the world, but in the context of the reasoning here, they may show that there is another more positive alternative to seeing the human as denying connectedness in complexity and only driven by self-interest. Simply said, we can understand that these 'windows on the world that are now presented in constant streams' may also trigger us morally in a positive motivational sense. The moral appeal of cosmopolitanism manifests thus in two ways: as a call for responsibility that we can no longer deny or escape from and also as a call for reflection and action that triggers our moral sense and motivation for engagement with the world.

In sum, the idea of connectedness in 'global complexity' thus inspires an understanding of cosmopolitanism as an 'awareness' of that complexity and, consequently, as a responsible attitude of reflexivity with regard to the own place, role, rights and responsibilities and specific interests, hopes, hypotheses, beliefs and concerns in that complexity. Obviously it makes no sense to only adopt that attitude in solitary reflection. The idea further developed in Meskens (2017) is that this kind of reflexivity may trigger a prepared-ness for rapprochement and engagement in deliberation with each other. The joint preparedness for 'public reflexivity' of all concerned participants would consequently enable a dialogue that, unavoidably, will also have a confron-tational character, as each would have to be prepared to give an account of his/her interests, hopes, hypotheses, beliefs and concerns with respect to the problem at stake. That joint preparedness can be described as a commitment to 'intellectual solidarity', as those concerned would have to be prepared to openly reflect with each other and towards the outside world about the way they not only rationalise the problem but also their own interests and the interests of others. From this simple but powerful insight flows the idea that if nobody has the full effective authority to make sense of a specific problem and its possible solutions, then participants have only each other as the (equal) points of references in deliberating on the problem. In 'The Ethical Project', the philosopher Philip Kitcher reflects to similar effect saying: 'there are no ethical experts' and that, therefore, authority can only be the authority of the conversation among the participants (Kitcher 2014).

Taken all this together, in terms of ethics, the idea of connectedness in 'global complexity' invites us to understand cosmopolitanism as the ethical attitude of reflexivity in face of the complexity of problems of a global scale and consequently as a sense for global intellectual solidarity and an ethi-cal commitment to seek rapprochement and engage in dialogue taking into account that global scale.[7] That meaning of cosmopolitanism is *identical* for every citizen of the world, which does obviously not mean, as already sug-gested before, that the practical implications are the same for all of us. Con-nectedness suggests a form of relational symmetry between subjects all over the world, but, understandably, place, role, rights and responsibilities mean different things for these subjects depending on their social and political sit-uation, standard of living and possibilities for self-realisation. We might all be 'citizens of the world' in terms of our responsibilities, but we also have our own specific capacities and vulnerabilities that influence not only our possibility to live a decent life but also the possibility to think and act as cosmopolitans.

As said before, the meaning and value of cosmopolitanism taking into account our various particular social situations will be taken up again at the end of this chapter. For now, as I here propose a specific meaning of the concept of cosmopolitanism, it is necessary to consider how it relates to other more traditional understandings of the concept. Contemporary discussions on cosmopolitanism – its conceptual meaning, the various arguments in favour or against, possible practical meanings – are diverse and fragmented, as well in academic context as in more informal public discourse. What the discussions have in common is that, in contrast to the early spiritual meanings referred to in section 2, contemporary conceptions of cosmopolitanism are normative in the way they motivate the idea based on critical evaluations of the real world today. In that sense, I think conceptions of cosmopolitanism can be situated in three categories:

1   Cosmopolitanism 'defined' on the basis of the promotion of values such as impartiality, equality and (global) justice;
2   Cosmopolitanism evaluated against contemporary politics and/or legal systems: identity politics, state-oriented politics, international law (e.g., in relation to the problem of forced migration);
3   Cosmopolitanism 'defined' as a 'stance' or 'attitude', or as a form of being and acting in the world.

Of course, grasping and describing the practical meaning of one specific category will inevitably result in relating it to the other two. The description of cosmopolitanism as the '… *demanding and contentious moral position that urges us to include the whole world in our moral concerns and to apply the standards of impartiality and equity across boundaries of nationality, race, religion and gender …*' (van Hooft 2009) may be of the most 'complete' in the way it refers to all three categories proposed above. A simple alternative is '*the view that the moral standing of all peoples and of each individual person around the globe is equal*' (van Hooft 2009). Important to note is the difference between these two understandings of cosmopolitanism: the first interprets the moral position as a commitment in response to an 'appeal from the world' comparable to the 'appeal of complexity' proposed above, while the second sounds more as an a priori commitment to equality as a fundamental value in itself. In addition, the first sounds as if others and the world 'depend' on our moral will to value inclusion, impartiality and equity, while the second 'declares' others as moral agents on 'equal footing' with ourselves. In other words, the first interpretation does not necessarily imply the second: one can still include the whole world in his/her moral concern and even apply the standards of impartiality and equity from out of some (self-acclaimed) moral superiority or technocratic paternalist position.

Despite of its simple form, the second understanding therefore feels as more all-encompassing, not only in its reciprocity but also because it specifically points at the importance of considering others as moral agents in themselves. Indeed, as the *Encyclopaedia Britannica* specifies,

> Moral standing, in ethics, [is] the status of an entity by virtue of which it is deserving of consideration in moral decision-making. To ask if an entity has moral standing is to ask whether the well-being of that entity should be taken into account by others; it is also to ask whether that entity has moral value or worth and whether it can make moral claims on other beings.
>
> (Encyclopaedia Britannica n.d.)

Taking the two understandings together, cosmopolitanism as a stance or attitude is thus the commitment to include the whole world in our moral concerns while considering each other in that world as of equal moral standing. However, this 'definition' does not specify what the consequences thereof are for the method of moral decision-making or what the required competences of everyone would need to be. In terms of competences, the first interpretation of cosmopolitanism above suggests at least that adopting this moral position is a demanding thing to do. As also van Hooft and Vandekerckhove argue,

> cosmopolitanism is not just about a new and expanded set of norms that apply to the global community. It is also about new ways of being: being a citizen of the world, being concerned for others who are distant strangers, and being committed to pursuing human rights and social justice anywhere in the world.
>
> (van Hooft and Vandekerckhove 2010)

In other words, according to this view, being a cosmopolitan requires us to not only reflect on moral issues and our own behaviour but also to engage in dialogue and to take action in the interest of 'pursuing human rights and social justice anywhere in the world'. The authors propose the concept of 'cosmopolitan subjectivity' as a subjectivity '… *lived by real people in concrete and normatively thick situations* …' (van Hooft and Vandekerckhove 2010, xvii), and this in contrast to the understanding of subjectivity from behind the Rawlsian 'veil of ignorance', abstracted from the own 'class position, social status and personal considerations' (Rawls 1971). From that perspective, van Hooft and Vandekerckhove list a series of 'cosmopolitanist attitudes' as aspects of these 'new ways of being'. In the interest of the reflections in this chapter, it is worthwhile to quote them in length on this:

> A cosmopolitan form of subjectivity differs in fundamental ways from the forms of subjectivity that express themselves in chauvinism, nationalism,

intolerance of difference, belligerence towards foreigners, racism, impe-
rialism, ignorance of other cultures, and bigotry. In our view, contemporary cosmopolitans evince a form of subjectivity that comprises all or
most of the following attitudes. They are suspicious of nationalism, all
forms of chauvinism, and even patriotism. They refuse to see the national
economic and military interests of their country as more important than
global values such as human rights, global justice and the protection of
the global environment, and they refuse to give their co-nationals any
priority in their concerns or responsibilities at the expense of more distant others. This is perhaps why they have earned the ire of nationalists
everywhere. They respect basic human rights, see them as universally
normative, and acknowledge the moral equality of all peoples and individuals. They consider the people of the world as united by reason,
sociability and a common humanity, and believe in a globally acceptable
concept of human dignity. In their actions they demonstrate benevolence
to all others irrespective of race, caste, nationality, religion, ethnicity or
location, and are willing to come to the aid of those suffering from natural or man-made disasters, including extreme poverty. They evince a
commitment to justice in the distribution of natural resources and wealth
on a global scale, and display solidarity with the struggles for human
rights and for social justice of all the world's peoples. They are happy for
the states of which they are citizens to open their borders to refugees and
immigrants and to embrace their differences into the national culture.
They long for, and work towards, lasting peace, and acknowledge the
rule of international law. They are opposed to tyranny and are committed to open and participatory political processes throughout the world.
They respect the right to self-determination of peoples. They display
tolerance of religious and cultural differences and accept the global existence of moral pluralism. They are prepared to enter into dialogue and
communication across cultural and national boundaries, and to see the
world as a single community.

(van Hooft and Vandekerckhove 2010, xvii–xviii)

How ultimately desirable this all sounds indeed, one can possibly agree the
authors go very far in describing the cosmopolitan as a kind of übermensch
capable of and committed to striving for 'all things good'. The authors do
however specify that '... *Such attitudes do not arise fully formed in the hearts and
minds of cosmopolitans. They need to be developed and nurtured through processes
of education and reflection...*' (van Hooft and Vandekerckhove 2010, xviii).
Analysis of the consequences thereof in literature on cosmopolitanism goes
beyond the scope of this chapter. More important here is a coupling back
of this view on cosmopolitanism to the idea of 'reflexivity in face of complexity', which I propose as a 'root attitude' of the cosmopolitan. First of all,
the exhaustive list of aspects of the cosmopolitans' moral attitude above may
also be read as a reference list of all the global challenges our society has to
deal with today. Second, one can understand that the required 'processes of

education and reflection' should not only concentrate on factual knowledge of these challenges but also and foremost on the 'nature' of their complexity (I refer to the reasoning from section 1 that they all have similar characteristics of complexity). However, my argument is that full insight in factual and normative complexity of these global challenges does not make you a cosmopolitan per se, unless that insight also triggers reflection with regard to one's own position in relation to these challenges. A sensitivity to the global complexity that binds us today, with the uncertainties, interlinkages and relative responsibilities that characterise the global problems we face, *may* trigger a moral sensitivity with regard to the value of impartiality and equity and with regard to the need to include the whole world in our moral concern, but that does not necessarily imply self-reflection with respect to our own 'rights and responsibilities' as a consequence. Only when we are prepared to reflect on our own position and behaviour 'in that whole world of concern' will we be able to see all other people as being of equal moral standing, simply because then we will not only see them as having equal moral standing in their own *right*, but because we can then consider them as also having equal moral *responsibility*. A cosmopolitan is thus not an übermensch capable of caring for all things good, but in the first place a human who thinks and acts from a reflexive position of *moral modesty* in that whole world of concern and who is *therefore* convinced that all (other) people are of equal moral standing.

Based on this reasoning, we are now able to formulate an understanding of what it means to be a cosmopolitan from the perspective of what it would imply to fairly deal with the complexity that binds us today, although using more traditional language on morality. In short, if we take as premises the 'fact of complexity' of our global social problems on the one hand, and the view that cosmopolitanism is the commitment to include the whole world in our moral concerns on the other, then the idea that we need to deal fairly with the complexity of these global problems makes us to understand cosmopolitanism as the preparedness

- to recognise the global complexity that binds us;
- to recognise our own 'moral modesty' in dealing with that global complexity and, thus, to recognise each other citizen of the world as being of equal moral standing;
- to recognise the importance of 'global intellectual solidarity' and, consequently, to seek rapprochement and to engage in deliberation with other citizens of the world.

The reader may note the similarity of this threefold 'preparedness' with the general conceptual understanding of reflexivity and intellectual solidarity suggested in Meskens (2017).[8] In other words, one could say that cosmopolitanism in relation to global complexity is the ideas of reflexivity as an ethical attitude and intellectual solidarity as an ethical commitment 'stretched to the global level'.

However, as it was already suggested before, the problem with this understanding is that it does not seem to take into account the fact that the possibility to think and act as a cosmopolitan depends on our social and political situation, standard of living and possibilities for self-realisation. This will be a point of attention in the next and concluding section of this chapter.

Cosmopolitanism as an ethics of care for environmental health

A preliminary reflection – on the politics of harmony (with nature)

One of the great tenets of Stoicism, the philosopher Anthony Clifford Grayling argues in the preface of Marcus Aurelius' Meditations, is that '*… whatever happens "in accordance with Nature" is for that very reason good, and that therefore the only bad things that can happen to people are the result of their own failings…*' (Marcus Aurelius 2002, preface by A.C. Grayling). Marcus Aurelius himself specified almost 2,000 years earlier that '*… Nothing can happen to any man that Nature has not fitted him to endure …*' (Marcus Aurelius 2002, Book V, statement 6) and that '*… All things come to their fulfilment as the one universal Nature directs …*' (Marcus Aurelius 2002, Book VI, statement 9). From his thoughts, we can understand that, for him, the idea of 'living in harmony with nature' for sure meant a harmony that nature itself directs and imposes on us as humble and vulnerable humans. If the UN now states that '*… it is necessary to promote Harmony with Nature in order to achieve a just balance among the economic, social and environmental needs of present and future generations …*' (United Nations n.d.) then we know we should understand their reference to nature the other way round: nature still in a way directs what harmony would mean, although now itself from out of the humble and vulnerable position originally destined to us humans.[9] The UN statement should also not be read as a call to go 'back to nature', on the contrary: the 'balance to strive for' is not a balance between humans and nature as such but the balance between our own economic, social and environmental needs, now and in the future. The 'just balance' refers to a morally right or fair balance of needs among humans (present and future), and nature is only instrumentally included in that moral concern. Critically interpreting the UN statement, harmony with nature thus means that we shouldn't harm it too much with our activities so that the consequences don't put our own (balanced) well-being in danger. Nature is not seen as an inseparable part of a whole to which we also belong, but as a backdrop and as a 'sustainable' resource and dump for our own activities.[10]

A preliminary reflection – on the (w)holism of complexity

In contrast to that actual political interpretation of harmony, the early cosmopolitans saw human beings as entities of 'an organic living whole, in which everything is related to everything else, and in which human individuals are "limbs" of the whole'. And, as Anthony Clifford Grayling said in the introduction to the Mediations, that meant that the well-being of individuals is dependent upon the well-being of everything else. Although this could be read as similar to the pragmatic understanding of harmony with nature expressed by the UN statement, we have to keep in mind that, for Marcus Aurelius and his other fellow cosmopolitans, living in that time meant 'living the way the one universal Nature directs'. So for them, holism, as the view that 'parts of a whole are interconnected such that they cannot exist independently of the whole, or cannot be understood without reference to the whole' was a holism directed by nature, not by humans.[11] While their view was spiritual and, as argued in section 2, 'not hindered by reality', today, a similar understanding of the concept of holism cannot escape taking into account that reality: not only do we humans have a considerable and observable impact on the state of our planet and on our own coexistence, the 'fact of complexity' also troubles the understanding of 'the parts in reference to the whole' and thus of the whole itself. In other words, holism can no longer be understood as a 'factual' interconnection between entities such as people, nature, acts, objects, phenomena and situations but as a holism that also has to take into account various factual and normative interpretations of these entities and their interconnections. Whether or not the early cosmopolitans thought the whole could in principle still be grasped and understood, for sure we can say this became impossible today. However, this should not be taken as a doomed reality, on the contrary. Rather than an invitation to fully 'know' the whole and the parts in relation to the whole, holism, in this 'new' meaning, is the awareness and insight that we are all bound in the complexity of that whole and that nature is bound with us. Precisely this situation should morally motivate us to seek rapprochement with the aim to try to 'know and understand together', and, for sure, this is a responsibility of us humans alone, as we cannot and should not include nature as an accountable partner. Paraphrasing what was said before, dealing fairly with each other in that whole implies a fair dealing with the complexity of influences and dependences that binds us within that whole. For the case of environmental health governance, that implies we should not only take into account 'aspects of the natural and built environment' of that whole but also and foremost the social, economic and political factors influencing ('affecting') these environments and the interpretations thereof.

Cosmopolitanism as an ethics of care (for each other's ethical competence)

Time to bring everything together. In the view on cosmopolitanism developed here, the recognition of the global complexity that binds us today stimulates reflexivity with regard to our own position, beliefs, interests, hopes, hypotheses and concerns in that global complexity, and, consequently, it stimulates the recognition of our own 'moral modesty' in dealing with that complexity. With the commitment to include the whole world in our moral concerns, that moral modesty not only motivates us to recognise each other citizen of the world as being of equal moral standing but also provides us with the insight that we *need* our fellow citizens and their moral opinions to make sense of that complexity. Based on that insight, cosmopolitans recognise the importance of 'global intellectual solidarity' and, consequently, the need to seek rapprochement and to engage in deliberation with other citizens of the world.

However, the reasoning does not end here. If cosmopolitans recognise other citizens as being of equal moral standing, then global intellectual solidarity does not only refer to our preparedness to engage in deliberation with each other in the world but also refer to our preparedness to care for each other's capability to engage in that deliberation. Capability can in this context be understood as comprising the 'practical' possibility for everyone to participate and also each other's intellectual and ethical competence to deliberate complex problems with their fellow citizens of the world. Cosmopolitanism as a theory can therefore essentially be considered as an ethics of care theory.[12] Caring for each other as cosmopolitans is also caring for each other's intellectual and ethical competence in order for everyone to be capable of reasoning from out of equal moral standing. Cosmopolitanism is therefore not only a personal 'cosmopolitanist attitude' while 'being in the world' but also a preparedness to care for the possibility of all citizens of the world to become ethically competent as cosmopolitans.

How to understand ethical competence in this context? Ethical competence could initially be understood as the ability to develop and 'use' an ethical sense or attitude with regard to ethical issues. As discussed before, in their book *Questioning Cosmopolitanism*, Van Hooft and Vandekerckhove argue that the list of 'cosmopolitanist attitudes' put forward by them 'don't arise fully formed in the hearts and minds of cosmopolitans' but rather 'need to be developed and nurtured through processes of education and reflection …' (van Hooft and Vandekerckhove 2010, xviii). In third section of this chapter, I added that a cosmopolitanist attitude would first and foremost need to be rooted in an attitude of reflexivity 'in face of complexity' (of particular issues and of the global complexity that binds us). Also this root cosmopolitanist attitude of reflexivity can be 'developed and nurtured through processes of education and reflection'. However, my proposal is that fair and effective governance of global complex problems in general, and of environmental health problems in particular, requires more than a cosmopolitan vision on education. I will end this chapter with a short reflection on this.

First of all, cosmopolitanism and its root attitude of reflexivity 'in face of global complexity' *can* be developed as ethical competences, but one can understand this should not be left to chance, depending on everyone's course of life. For sure, the world leisure traveller, the United Nations Volunteer,[13] the climate change refugee[14] and the poor farmer coping with land degradation may individually develop some kind of 'cosmopolitanist experience', being confronted with globalisation in general and with specific environmental health issues in particular, but one can understand that these experiences are far from comparable and trigger the ethical sense in different ways. The traveller may satisfy their curiosity and develop a respect for nature and other cultures, and the volunteer, driven by a social engagement, may develop insight into the complexity of local situations and their interlinkages with the global, but one can say both of them enjoy specific possibilities – in the sense of *capabilities* – to voluntarily develop these 'cosmopolitanist attitudes'. Their 'right to be responsible' as cosmopolitan is ensured by their capability and freedom to use that right. The refugee and the farmer, on the other hand, are affected by global environmental health problems that hinder them in even living a practical decent life. Overthinking their difficult situation will for sure trigger their ethical sense, but the suggestion that we all would need to think and act as cosmopolitans will be the least of their daily concerns. Their grim situation is not only undermining their health and general well-being; it is also denying their right to be responsible as intrinsically capable citizens of the world.

The stories of the world leisure traveller, the UN Volunteer, the climate change refugee and the poor farmer support the view that, if caring for each other as cosmopolitans is caring for each other's equal possibilities to think and act as cosmopolitans, this 'care perspective' first and foremost needs to consider everyone's sociopolitical situation, standard of living, and possibilities for self-realisation.[15] Important to note here is that, from out of a cosmopolitanist ethics of care perspective, our standards of living and sociopolitical situations don't necessarily need to be the same or 'equal' to enable ourselves to develop, think and act as cosmopolitans. The essential concern of the cosmopolitanist ethics of care perspective proposed here is the striving for equality of our possibilities – again in the sense of capabilities – for self-realisation, given that these capabilities could in their turn positively influence our sociopolitical situation and standard of living. This vision on well-being is also the central idea of the well-known Capability Approach,[16] although the reader may understand that I aim to reinterpret that idea here away from the economic basis for well-being and with a focus on our capabilities to become (self-)critical and ethically competent world citizens. The essential idea is that there is no straightforward 'procedure' to 'produce' these cosmopolitans. For all of us, developing and 'using' the ethical competences of cosmopolitanism and its root attitude of reflexivity essentially happens through the 'ethical experience' of interacting with others. This 'cosmopolitan experience' may happen informally and coincidentally in the course of our lives, but the examples above show that, as a form of social justice, it should also be made possible for everyone through formal interaction methods and processes that enable and stimulate this experience. The 'root' interaction method is a pluralist, inclusive and transdisciplinary education that would enable everyone to become a (self-)critical world citizen; the other essential method is a form of democracy based on inclusion aiming, in the words of the American pragmatist philosopher John Dewey, to 'socialize' the intelligence of the people (see Dewey and Tufts 1908; Gouinlock 1994, among others). In other words, a cosmopolitanist method of negotiation and decision-making inspired by the ethical attitudes of reflexivity and intellectual solidarity would be inclusive, deliberative and democratic. It would see deliberation as a collective self-critical reflection and learning process among all concerned, rather than as a competition between conflicting views driven by self-interest. Important to note for democratic deliberation is that, in a cosmopolitan ethics of care perspective, these methods and processes don't need themselves to be global in scale per se. Cosmopolitan deliberative dialogues can be organised in every setting, from a local village to nationally bound democracies to the global level of negotiations facilitated by the UN. With regard to the last, it is relevant to emphasize that, different from the UN Resolution on 'Harmony with Nature', the development of the Earth Charter was a worldwide civil society initiative. An independent Earth Charter Commission was formed in 1997 to oversee the development of the text, analyse the outcomes of a worldwide consultation process and to come to an agreement on a global consensus document (The Earth Charter n.d.). Important in this context is that its first article also hints at the idea of 'capabilities' for environmental health from the same holistic perspective:

> 1. Respect Earth and life in all its diversity.
> – Recognize that all beings are interdependent and every form of life has value regardless of its worth to human beings.
> – Affirm faith in the inherent dignity of all human beings and in the intellectual, artistic, ethical, and spiritual potential of humanity.
>
> (The Earth Charter n.d. Article 1)

Conclusion – cosmopolitanism as a human right?

In this chapter, I argued that environmental health problems are global complex problems that require a cosmopolitan perspective and approach. I proposed a specific cosmopolitan ethics of care perspective and briefly reflected on how a cosmopolitan experience and dialogue could be put in practice. A further reflection on how this could and should effectively be organised and what kind of political reform towards this goal would be needed is essential but beyond the scope of this chapter. Another ethical issue of further concern is a cosmopolitan ethics of care perspective on our responsibility towards the future generations. In principle, cosmopolitans also include the future world in their moral concern and see their future fellow citizens as being of equal moral standing. We cannot and should not try to control how these future cosmopolitans would approach environmental health problems themselves, but we can do a lot today. As cosmopolitans, we have the possibility to care for our global intragenerational relationships and to care for cosmopolitan capabilities of our next generation. In addition to that, the 'only' thing we can and should do more is to explain the far future why we thought – together – this was the best thing we could do.

Finally, let's phrase the ideas proposed here the other way round: do we all need to (be able to) think and act as cosmopolitans in the interest of fair and effective environmental health governance? The answer 'yes', underpinned with reasonable argument and reflection, as I aimed to do here, can be called an informed opinion, but it is obviously not supported by a convincing proof. But that is not the point. What would be interesting is to hear informed opinions on why we *wouldn't* need a cosmopolitan perspective and a care for related methods and capabilities in this respect. Concerns over practical feasibilities are important, but, in my opinion, they cannot be used to relativise the ethical perspective as such. Already today, cosmopolitan dialogues in the interest of environmental health governance can be organised everywhere and on every level and scale. They don't need a priori political reform of education and democracy but can, in their own way, inspire and stimulate that reform. Cosmopolitanism as an ethics of care that includes the whole world in its concern is essentially an ethics of care towards the individual human being. Our responsibilities as cosmopolitan human beings lean on our capabilities to understand the practical and ethical consequences of our acts and to reason on our specific place, role, responsibilities and rights in the bigger picture. Therefore, becoming a cosmopolitan, ethically competent to contribute to dealing with issues such as environmental health, is not only a responsibility but also everyone's human right.

Notes

1 I wrote about the 'justice of justification' of technological risk in general, and of radiological risk in particular, in Meskens (2016).
2 It may be clear that globalisation, as a trend or 'situation', refers to more than only our socioeconomic practices. Travel and communication now span the complete globe, and, together with the global market dynamic, all this has resulted in a 'global culture' marked by homogenisation and gentrification. Also disasters and risks (such as that of climate change and the Covid-19 pandemic) and the politics of war now have global dimensions. Last but not least, there is the impact of culture on politics leading to tensions on global scale, often characterised as a 'conflict between civilisations' or as a 'divide' between modern liberal societies and traditional theocracies. With all these dynamics playing on a global scale, also international diplomacy dealing with these dynamics became global in its scope and activity (adapted from van Hooft 2009).
3 Land degradation is probably one of the lesser known global environmental health problems. The Global Environment Facility (GEF) defines it as '… *the deterioration or loss of the productive capacity of the soils for present and future …*'. According to the GEF, '… *Globally, about 25 percent of the total land area has been degraded …*'. It further specifies that '… *When land is degraded, soil carbon and nitrous oxide is released into the atmosphere, making land degradation one of the most important contributors to climate change. Scientists recently warned that 24 billion tons of fertile soil was being lost per year, largely due to unsustainable agriculture practices. If this trend continues, 95 percent of the Earth's land areas could become degraded by 2050 …*' (Global Environment Facility 2016).

4 I wrote about the idea of dealing fairly with the complexity of complex social problems and about reflexivity as an ethical attitude and intellectual solidarity as ethical commitment 'in face of complexity' (Meskens 2017).

5 See, for instance, Fuchs (2018) for a general critical analysis of the adverse effects of 'digital capitalism' and Sánchez de la Sierra (2019) for the special case of the coltan mines in Eastern Congo.

6 According to the Buddhist thinker Matthieu Ricard, 'real' altruism is a mental attitude, motivation and intention (Ricard 2015). However, one can understand that acting upon that attitude, motivation and intention will only have a limited and temporal effect if at the same time cultures of paternalism, technocracy and conservatism curtail our possibility to engage in practice. Also, altruism as a 'mental attitude' is of course not a typical Buddhist perspective. Since the concept was proposed by the French philosopher Auguste Comte, the meaning of altruism and the motivations for altruism as an 'attitude' have been the topic of study in philosophy as well as in (evolutionary) psychology and evolutionary biology. For the latter, see, among others, Wilson (2015).

7 An ethical commitment to seek rapprochement and engage in dialogue taking into account the global scale is one thing, and caring for a dialogue on a global scale is another. The understanding of cosmopolitanism as proposed here includes the preparedness in principle to organise that dialogue on a global scale, taking into account the practical possibilities of and hindrances to doing so. A cosmopolitan could in that sense support the dialogues facilitated by the UN while still being sceptical about their democratic quality and effectiveness.

8 In Meskens (2017), I proposed that dealing fairly with the complexity of complex social problems requires the joint preparedness of all concerned to adopt a three-fold responsible attitude, identical for all concerned:

   a   The preparedness to recognise the complexity of complex social problems;
   b   (following a) The preparedness to acknowledge the imperative character of that complexity or thus to acknowledge one's own 'authority problem' in making sense of that complexity;
   c   (following b) The preparedness to recognise the importance of intellectual solidarity and, consequently, to seek rapprochement and engage in deliberation with other concerned participants.

9 The idea of the need to live in harmony with nature existed already longer in UN context. UNGA Resolution 64/196 of 2009 refers itself to Resolution 35/7 from 1980 on a 'Draft World Charter for Nature', stating, among other things, that '… *life on earth is part of nature and depends on the uninterrupted functioning of natural systems* …' and that '… *the benefits which can be obtained from nature depend on the maintenance of natural processes and on the diversity of life-forms and that those benefits are jeopardized by the excessive exploitation and the destruction of natural habitats* …' (UNGA 1980). Since then, one could possibly detect a more human- and society-centred evolution of the interpretation of harmony with nature taking more the position of a backdrop. A further discussion on this is beyond the scope of this chapter.

10 The view in which nature in general, and its living species and even 'objects' (such as a stone) in particular, are vulnerable but have moral standing in themselves is central to various 'rights of nature' theories and activist positions. A discussion of these would lead us too far in the context of this chapter, although one reflection is relevant here: we might (spiritually or symbolically) consider nature as having equal moral standing in its own *right*, but we can never assign it *responsibility*. Therefore, as humans, our responsibility could be called a 'responsible anthropocentrism' towards other humans and towards nature, the last not as a means but as an end in itself.

11 Important to note here however is that although the views of the early cosmopolitans could be understood as 'holistic', the word 'holism' only emerged in

modern times. It was first proposed by Jan Christiaan Smuts – a South African and British Commonwealth statesman, British field marshal in the Second World War, and philosopher – in his book *Holism and Evolution*. Interestingly enough, he still used it as referring to nature, saying that holism is 'the tendency in nature to form wholes that are greater than the sum of the parts through creative evolution' (Smuts 1926).

12 'Ethics of care' is an ethics theory that seeks reference in the care for human relationships. The problem with this theory is that it might 'work' for close relations with known people (such as in families and between friends or in medical context between doctor, patient and relatives of the patient) but that it remains unclear how it could work for distant relations with strangers. In Meskens (2017), I argued that the vision that we are all 'bound in complexity' can inspire an ethics of care for those distant relations with strangers. The idea that 'we are all in it together' informs the view that we should care for our relations with each other, not only in the sense that we need to be reflexive with respect to how our complex relations 'emerge' and 'work' but also in the sense that we need each other to make sense of the complexity that binds us.

13 The United Nations Volunteers (UNV) programme aims to contribute to peace and development through facilitating volunteerism worldwide (United Nations Volunteers n.d.)

14 The Global Compact on Refugees, adopted by the UNGA in December 2018, recognises that 'climate, environmental degradation and natural disasters increasingly interact with the drivers of refugee movements' (United Nations Refugee Agency n.d.).

15 In that sense, the authors Bruce Robbins and Paulo Lemos Horta propose the idea that 'there is more than one kind of cosmopolitanism' and that cosmopolitanism, instead of interpreting it as 'one single ideal against which all smaller loyalties and forms of belonging are judged', can be defined as 'one of many possible modes of life, thought and sensibility that are produced when commitments and loyalties are multiple and overlapping' (Robbins and Horta 2017). The authors link the concept of cosmopolitanisms (plural) to the idea of 'belonging' to specific 'sociohistorical sites and situations of multiple membership'. Their interpretation of the concept thus starts from a different perspective than the one used by van Hooft and Vandekerckhove and the one I propose here. An elaboration on how this interpretation is not in contradiction but could rather work complementary and enriching is beyond the scope of this chapter.

16 The capability approach is essentially an economics theory introduced by the economist-philosopher Amartya Sen and further developed by philosopher Martha Nussbaum and a growing number of other scholars across the humanities and the social sciences. As the *Stanford Encyclopedia of Philosophy* puts it,

> The capability approach is a theoretical framework that entails two core normative claims: first, the claim that the freedom to achieve well-being is of primary moral importance, and second, that freedom to achieve well-being is to be understood in terms of people's capabilities, that is, their real opportunities to do and be what they have reason to value.
>
> (Robeyns 2016)

References

Appiah, Kwame Anthony. 2015. *Cosmopolitanism: Ethics in a World of Strangers*. Penguin Books, London, England.

Busscher, Nienke, Eva Lia Colombo, Lidewij van der Ploeg, Julia Inés Gabella, and Amalia Leguizamón. 2020. 'Civil Society Challenges the Global Food System:

The International Monsanto Tribunal'. *Globalizations* 17 (1): 16–30. https://doi.or g/10.1080/14747731.2019.1592067.

Carrington, Damian. 2020. 'Halt Destruction of Nature or Suffer Even Worse Pandemics, Say World's Top Scientists'. *The Guardian*. April 2020. http://www.theguardian.com/ world/2020/apr/27/halt-destruction-nature-worse-pandemics-top-scientists.

Dewey, John, and James H. Tufts. 1908. *Ethics*. USA: University of California Libraries.

Encyclopaedia Britannica. n.d. 'Moral Standing | Ethics'. Encyclopaedia Britannica. 23 June 2020. https://www.britannica.com/topic/moral-standing.

Fuchs, Christian. 2018. 'Capitalism, Patriarchy, Slavery, and Racism in the Age of Digital Capitalism and Digital Labour'. *Critical Sociology* 44 (4–5): 677–702. https:// doi.org/10.1177/0896920517691108.

Global Environment Facility. 2016. 'Land Degradation'. Global Environment Facility. 24 March 2016. https://www.thegef.org/topics/land-degradation.

Gouinlock, James. 1994. *The Moral Writings of John Dewey*. Rev Sub edition. US: Prometheus Books.

Hooft, Stan van. 2009. *Cosmopolitanism: A Philosophy for Global Ethics*. McGill-Queen's University Press Canada. https://www.jstor.org/stable/j.ctt7zt1fm.

Hooft, Stan van, and Wim Vandekerckhove, eds. 2010. *Questioning Cosmopolitanism*. 2011 edition. Dordrecht; New York: Springer.

Kitcher, Philip. 2014. *The Ethical Project*. Cambridge, MA: Harvard University Press.

Liu, Xiaojun, Hui Zhu, Yongxin Hu, Sha Feng, Yuanyuan Chu, Yanyan Wu, Chiyu Wang, Yuxuan Zhang, Zhaokang Yuan, and Yuanan Lu. 2016. 'Public's Health Risk Awareness on Urban Air Pollution in Chinese Megacities: The Cases of Shanghai, Wuhan and Nanchang'. *International Journal of Environmental Research and Public Health* 13 (9): 845. https://doi.org/10.3390/ijerph13090845.

Marcus Aurelius. 2002. *Meditations*. Reprint edition, from The original translation by Maxwell Staniforth for Penguin Books Ltd. 1964. UK: The Folio Society.

Meskens, Gaston. 2016. 'Ethics of Radiological Risk Governance: Justice of Justification as a Central Concern'. *Annals of the ICRP* 45 (1 Suppl.): 322–344. https:// doi.org/10.1177/0146645316639837.

———. 2017. 'Better Living (in a Complex World): An Ethics of Care for Our Modern Co-Existence'. In *Ethics of Environmental Health* (pp. 115–136), edited by Zölzer, Friedo & Meskens, Gaston. Routledge Studies in Environment and Health. UK: Routledge.

Peschard, Karine, and Shalini Randeria. 2020. 'Taking Monsanto to Court: Legal Activism around Intellectual Property in Brazil and India'. *The Journal of Peasant Studies* 47 (4): 792–819. https://doi.org/10.1080/03066150.2020.1753184.

Rawls, John. 1971. *A Theory of Justice*. Revised Edition 1999. Cambridge, MA: The Belknap Press of Harvard University Press.

Ricard, Matthieu. 2015. Altruism: The Power of Compassion to Change Yourself and the World. Tra edition. New York, NY: Little, Brown and Company.

Robbins, Bruce, and Paulo Lemos Horta, eds. 2017. *Cosmopolitanisms*. Reprint edition. New York: NYU Press.

Robeyns, Ingrid. 2016. 'The Capability Approach'. In *The Stanford Encyclopedia of Philosophy*, edited by Edward N. Zalta. USA: Metaphysics Research Lab, Stanford University. https://plato.stanford.edu/archives/win2016/entries/capability-approach/.

Rodwin, Victor G., and Michael K. Gusmano. 2002. 'The World Cities Project: Rationale, Organization, and Design for Comparison of Megacity Health Systems'. *Journal of Urban Health* 79 (4): 445. https://doi.org/10.1093/jurban/79.4.445.

Sánchez de la Sierra, Raúl. 2019. 'On the Origins of the State: Stationary Bandits and Taxation in Eastern Congo'. *Journal of Political Economy* 128 (1): 32–74. https://doi.org/10.1086/703989.

Smuts, Jan Christiaan. 1926. *Holism and Evolution*. USA: Macmillan Inc.

Stone, Madeleine. 2020. 'A Plague of Locusts Has Descended on East Africa. Climate Change May Be to Blame.' *Science*. 14 February 2020. https://www.nationalgeographic.com/science/2020/02/locust-plague-climate-science-east-africa/.

The Earth Charter. n.d. 'Earth Charter | Turning Conscience into Action for a Thriving Earth'. 14 April 2020. https://earthcharter.org/.

United Nations. n.d. 'Harmony with Nature'. 10 April 2020. http://www.harmonywithnatureun.org/.

United Nations General Assembly. 1980. 'Resolution 35/7 Draft World Charter for Nature'. United Nations. https://undocs.org/en/A/RES/35/7.

———. 2009. 'Resolution Adopted by the General Assembly on 21 December 2009, [on the Report of the Second Committee (A/64/420)], 64/196. Harmony with Nature'. United Nations. https://undocs.org/A/RES/64/196.

United Nations Refugee Agency. n.d. 'Climate Change and Disaster Displacement'. UNHCR. 11 September 2020. https://www.unhcr.org/climate-change-and-disasters.html.

United Nations Volunteers. n.d. 'UNV | VOLUNTEERS'. 11 September 2020. https://www.unv.org/.

Wikipedia. 2020. 'Environmental Health'. *Wikipedia*. https://en.wikipedia.org/w/index.php?title=Environmental_health&oldid=949831659.

Wilson, David Sloan. 2015. *Does Altruism Exist? Culture, Genes, and the Welfare of Others*. New Haven, CT; London: Yale University Press.

World Health Organisation. 2020. 'Urgent Health Challenges for the Next Decade'. 13 January 2020. https://www.who.int/news-room/photo-story/photo-story-detail/urgent-health-challenges-for-the-next-decade.

———. n.d. 'Constitution'. 10 August 2020. https://www.who.int/about/who-we-are/constitution.

Zölzer, Friedo, and Gaston Meskens, eds. 2017. *Ethics of Environmental Health*. UK: Routledge. http://hdl.handle.net/1854/LU-8555283.

———, eds. 2019. *Environmental Health Risks: Ethical Aspects*. 1st edition. UK: Routledge.

Part 2

Ethical challenges in toxicological research

4 Toward a medico-legal convergence to ethically protect the public's health

Carl F. Cranor

Chronic diseases, displacing infectious diseases, have become the major threat to good health in developed countries. This chapter considers two broadly different legal approaches to reducing chronic diseases caused by environmental toxicants and some major ethical issues of these institutions and scientific research in support of them against the background of other health protections. The argument pursues four main points. (1) Chronic diseases are of concern to physicians, to environmental health scientists, and to researchers who seek to prevent them from befalling the broader public. Prevention of such diseases is important because they are typically accompanied by numerous morbidities—debilitating conditions—that interfere with our lives. (2) Physicians' concern with the "primordial prevention" of chronic diseases sets an important ethical standard for using science to prevent risks that lead to diseases and provides a model to which other institutions should reasonably aspire. (3) Recent scientific findings revealing the origins of disease during development and the significance of vulnerabilities to disease from toxic substances at other periods of life greatly increase the urgency to adopt primordial prevention to protect children, the broader public, and the workforce. (4) Throughout I note a variety of ethical and normative choices that permeate different strategies for health protection and scientific research in support of better protections. This reveals substantial cognitive dissonance between different institutions that seek to protect people's health. Ethically we should seek better convergence between physicians' and our concern to have good health and community institutions that often fail to protect it.

Background

For centuries, infectious diseases, plagues, and pandemics afflicted humans. However, with environmental cleanup, increased biological understanding of bacteria and viruses, and the development of antibiotics and vaccines about a century ago developed countries began to control the infectious ravages of previous centuries. Public health officials removed horses' manure from streets and cleaned up sewage in rivers, major sources of diseases. They also chlorinated drinking water, while researchers developed antibiotics, and

DOI: 10.4324/9780429318436-7

discovered and used vaccines to prevent diseases, substantially reducing infectious diseases.

However, in the developed world, chronic diseases have become the leading causes of morbidity and mortality (Fries, 1980; Wigle and Lanphear, 2005). These maladies can be quite serious and long-lived and include cancers, neurological disorders, immune dysfunctions, lung diseases, diabetes, and cardiovascular diseases. They are not "prevented by vaccines, [typically are not] cured by medication," are "not communicable … and do not just disappear" (MedicineNet). Chronic diseases also typically exhibit a number of morbidities: ongoing congestive heart failure, diabetes, asthma, chronic obstructive pulmonary disorder, arthritis, or conditions after the first heart attacks that hamper age-specific good health (Fries et al., 2011; Dietert et al., 2010).

The morbidities of chronic diseases, not easy to eliminate, can cause substantial interference with a person's life-long normal good health and flourishing (Fries, 1980). However, access to health care and physicians' guidance can modify the prognosis or lessen the effects of some conditions, for example, "[t[reatment of hypertension retards development of certain complications in the arteries" (Fries et al., 1980). Physicians also urge patients to modify their behavior to prevent or reduce the risks that lead to the onset of these diseases, which in turn could compress *the period during which persons might experience morbidity*. Fries et al. (2011), ethically concerned about their patients, recommend four preventive steps to postpone or reduce chronic diseases and their lifetime morbidities.

> (1) "Primordial" Prevention prevents the *risk factor* (not the illness) from developing. For instance, decreasing the number of teenagers who start smoking or preventing childhood obesity represents primordial prevention; (2) *Primary Prevention* decreases risk factor prevalence, as by stopping smoking, promoting exercise, reducing weight, and reducing hypertension and cholesterol levels; (3) *Secondary Prevention* is aimed at preventing progression of disease, as in decreasing second heart attacks, congestive heart failure, or complications of diabetes; (4) *Tertiary Prevention* aims at reduction of morbid states that have already occurred, as with replacement of faulty hips, failed kidneys or livers, or use of a scooter for locomotion. Tertiary Prevention can … but often does not eliminate [morbidity]. A strategic approach to reduction in lifetime morbidity requires all four approaches … [summarized in Table 4.1].
>
> (Fries et al., 2011)

"Primordial prevention" is preferred because it prevents a risk factor, a potential source of disease, which helps postpone "most of the morbidity in life into a shorter period with less lifetime disability" (Fries et al., 2011). As people age bodily organs lose their reserves and the body tends to "rust out," rather than "wear out." They also propose, "If loss of reserve function represents aging in some sense, then exercising an organ presents a strategy for modifying the

Table 4.1 Examples of preventive medical strategies

Medical-personal	Primordial prevention— *prevent the risk factor from developing*	Primary prevention— *decrease the risk factor prevalence; stop the source of risks*	Secondary prevention— *prevent the progression of disease*	Tertiary prevention— *reduce morbid states that have already occurred with treatment*
Lung disease, emphysema, COPD	Never smoke	Quit smoking early in life	Reduce, quit smoking later if not earlier	Surgery, other treatment
Diabetes, atherosclerosis	Never become obese	Reduce obesity/ increase exercise	Reduce cholesterol, hypertension, extend time to first heart attack	Heart surgery, stents, statins
Diabetes, atherosclerosis	Avoid sedentary behavior; exercise your body	Begin exercise	Begin exercise later if not earlier	Diabetes treatment
Liver disease, cirrhosis	Don't drink to excess/ at all?	Quit the habit	Quit later if not earlier	Treat adverse conditions; possibly receive a liver transplant

aging process" (Fries et al., 2011). Thus, they urge individuals to adopt personal habits to promote their own health and to forestall the risk and "rust" of chronic diseases. Good health habits can lead "to greatly increased functional ability, decreased lifetime disability, and longer lives, with effects on morbidity greater than those upon mortality" (Fries et al., 2011).

There are sterling examples of people who implicitly or explicitly have avoided chronic diseases and followed life plans during various life stages, continuing to flourish when others chose rocking chairs. These include the oldest people to climb Africa's highest mountain, Kilimanjaro, or to climb Mt. Everest at the age of 73 (the oldest woman) or 80 (the oldest man), and many others. A 105-year-old cyclist is both improving his cycling speed and increasing his capacity to utilize oxygen at an age when such capacities typically wane.

Chronic diseases have a number of sources: bad luck, unfortunate genes, voluntary behavior, and the actions of others. The major, but not the only, focus of what follows is how administrative laws assisted by science can reduce chronic diseases that are caused by others. Physicians' concern for their patients' good health provides an ethical model from which we can learn. If physicians urge primordial prevention from the risks of disease, should not community health-protective institutions seek to prevent or reduce to the risks of chronic diseases caused by others and similarly endorse primordial prevention of risks? The science used in support of environmental health laws should also aim at identifying and primordially preventing risks of disease.

Toxic substances also contribute to chronic diseases

Exposures to toxic substances can also trigger chronic diseases, such as neurological diseases or dysfunctions; immune system disorders; cancer; lung diseases, such as coronary-artery disease or chronic obstructive pulmonary disease (COPD); and some diabetes (Cranor, 2011). Personal choices typically have a quite limited role in reducing risks from the vast majority of toxicants—cigarette smoking and excessive drinking aside. Rather, disease prevention must be pursued with the law.

Consider the example of Brian Milward who worked as a refrigerator repairman, using a number of fluids that contained the well-known carcinogen benzene as a solvent. His benzene exposure from 22 different products at age 47 surprised him with the disease, acute promyelocytic leukemia (APL) (Eastmond, 2012; *Milward v. Acuity Specialty Products, Inc.*, 2011). This occurs in only about one person per million in the U.S. population annually. However, because of his disease, chemotherapy, and associated conditions, at age 57 he was left "with 'absolutely ridiculous' fatigue" (Lombardi, 2014). Poor health forced him to retire early and take disability. His career and lifetime opportunities were greatly diminished: He could not do what he loves: repair racecars, work in his yard, play with his grandchildren. "It just sucks when you get a cancer like this" (Lombardi, 2014).

Milward's disease and its treatment not only truncated his life-long opportunities, but other citizens created the products containing benzene that curtailed his opportunities. He was treated doubly unjustly: A toxic ingredient, benzene, known to cause APL (Myron, 1992), in products created by others caused his disease and truncated his opportunities. Institutions permitted these harmful outcomes: Companies created products, likely using insufficient or no science to understand the risks, probably poorly testing them for adverse health effects because the law did not sufficiently control exposures. In addition, it seems no one and no institution sufficiently assessed the risks from multiple benzene exposures from different products, which led to his disease (*Milward v. Acuity Specialty Products*, 2011). For example, Milward's employer would have used different products in his business had he understood some of them contained benzene.

Contrast Brian Milward's fate with the sterling examples of others (noted above) who had quite good health at surprising and advanced ages with their periods of morbidity substantially postponed. Of course, people do not have to be world-class athletes to live long and prosper, as Dr. Spock of Star Trek endorsed, but it helps. Good health fosters a full and robust human life. We should all hope for this, and Fries et al., (2011) show how individuals can contribute to their own good health.

However, should we not collectively demand in areas of our lives, in which personal choices do not control our health but community institutions do, that these institutions also protect us from chronic diseases? In 1971, the U.S. President's Council on Environmental Quality at the beginnings of the environmental movement implicitly recognized this approach: "We should no longer be limited to repairing the damage after it has been done [a reference to the tort law]; nor should we continue to allow the entire population or the entire environment to be used as a laboratory" (U.S. Council on Environmental Quality, 1971). The Council urged for creating an improved standard for public health laws accompanied by appropriate science, but ethically our legislative and other institutions failed to act on this recommendation.

A justice case for preventing chronic diseases

Why is good health important for the populace? It provides an important foundation for an individual's good life and well-functioning in the community. It has been anecdotally clear during debates about access to health care in the United States that people greatly value it. More systematically, the ethical importance of protecting health with community institutions has been highlighted by the significance of health protection and health care implied by the most important theory of justice in the last 100 years—John Rawls' *A Theory of Justice* (1999) (Daniels, 1981; Cranor, 2011, 2017).

Rawls, followed by others, articulates two fundamental justice concerns that support health protections and health care. Aspects of his first principle of justice capture one idea: Each person should have an equal right to the most extensive freedom from physical assault (part of integrity of the person) compatible with a like freedom for all (Rawls, 1999). Invading toxicants are physical, but invisible assaulting substances, and many of them can cause harm through chronic diseases.

With extensions, Rawls's fair equality of opportunity principle (FEOP) reinforces the ethical import of preventing harm from toxicants and securing good health (Daniels, 1981; Cranor, 2017). Both principles ethically point to why good health is so important. It is quite significant to prevent chronic diseases because of their seriousness and their accompanying morbidities that can be intrusive, harmful, and unpleasant, often for much of a lifetime.

A rationale for FEOP is that every country (developed or less developed) has a range of opportunities for its citizens depending upon its wealth, technological and industrial advances, education, natural resources, and so on. It has long been settled that it is unjust to erect legal barriers to opportunities that, for example, forbid women, disfavored minorities, or those with particular religions from pursuing life goals compatible with their talents, abilities, and motivations (Rawls, 1999). However, there are also subtler barriers to opportunities, and reasons of justice support the idea that community institutions should not arbitrarily disadvantage an individual from pursuing his or her opportunities consistent with that person's talents, abilities, and motivation, although some will be more fortunate and some less fortunate in the distribution of these qualities (Daniels, 1981; Rawls, 1999). This principle recognizes the equal status and standing of each person in the community. In recognizing the equal status of each person in a just society, community institutions should secure as best they can that no person should be arbitrarily precluded by the basic institutions of society, including health care and health protection institutions, from pursuing opportunities consistent with that person's talents, abilities, and motivations (Daniels, 1981; Rawls, 1999; Cranor, 2017).

Consider how serious diseases can undermine opportunities. Chronic diseases caused by exposures to toxicants can interrupt and derail one's life in haphazard, unexpected, arbitrary, and serious ways, and often persisting for long periods of time. Children may come down with childhood cancer, asthma, lead poisoning, or some form of mental retardation. Adults may contract diabetes, cancer, mesothelioma, chronic obstructive lung disease, or thyroid disease; suffer a stroke, heart attack, or Parkinson's disease; or develop immune system disorders. Combined health protection and health care institutions can prevent or reduce many of these diseases and counteract haphazard disease-created opportunity barriers.

These considerations highlight the ethical importance of community health protection and health care institutions. I consider administrative laws that seek to address and prevent ethically random opportunity disadvantages that may arise from the lottery of diseases by focusing in particular on environmental and workplace maladies.[1] A just health protection and health care system would have institutions to prevent and treat diseases at different life stages and ages—prenatally and postnatally, during the years of development to adulthood, through a typically healthy mid-life, and into old age (Cranor, 2016, 2017; Heindel, 2018).

The law's contribution to a lifetime arc of good health and flourishing

Administrative health agencies, created by laws authorizing administrators to implement legal protections, ethically should be one of the main institutions to legally prevent (or at least substantially reduce) toxicity-caused chronic diseases. Legislators have ethical choices in how these laws are designed: Will they create laws well in order to achieve protective outcomes? Have they done so (Cranor, 2017)? Merely writing laws does not ensure their success. They must also be administered well and supported by ethically produced science to provide protections. I argue below that postmarket laws have fallen quite short on these dimensions, indicating some contrasts with premarket approval laws.

Personal injury (or the tort) law provides a venue in which people can be compensated for diseases caused by the products or conduct of others, but I do not consider the tort law here (Cranor, 2017).

How well have administrative laws functioned? When have they not functioned well? Why have there been shortcomings? How could they function better to more closely achieve primordial prevention of diseases?

Administrative laws

Two broadly different administrative strategies address diseases caused by toxic substances.

(1) Under U.S. laws for *pharmaceuticals* (1962) and *pesticides* (1968) Congress, perhaps understanding something of the importance of primordial risk prevention, ethically chose to place high priority on using science under these laws to test substances and understand any potential risks *before people are exposed*. They require *prudent testing* for possible risks of disease in general and also risks of disease that might be triggered by the specific chemical in question before the public is exposed to the products. Call these *premarket* testing and approval laws (Cranor, 2017).

For instance, a new pharmaceutical can only be approved for use if its health benefits outweigh its health risks. A company must conduct some preclinical testing to ensure that there are no undue risks to research subjects on whom the drug would be tested later. Companies must include information about chemical characteristics, pharmacological and toxicological information from animals, and in vitro systems along with a plan of clinical studies. Animal carcinogenicity studies must be conducted on products that would be administered chronically to a large population. If a product passes these tests, it then typically goes through three increasingly larger clinical trials with people to assess its effectiveness and safety that are reviewed by independent scientists. If it satisfactorily passes these studies and approved for commercialization, a large epidemiological study may need to be subsequently conducted to ensure that it is appropriately safe for large, genetically heterogeneous populations (U.S. Congress, Office of Technology Assessment, 1987). Central to laws for pharmaceuticals appears to be something approaching primordial prevention of disease risks from approved drugs.

I should note that the best health protections are provided by the structure of U.S. laws for pharmaceuticals and the *needed science in support of them*. This is not to suggest that all premarket laws should have the same requirements. The premarket pesticide laws require different science to try to ensure that pesticides are appropriately safe. Laws for general chemicals certainly need not require the kinds of scientific tests as are used for pharmaceuticals (because general chemicals are not designed to be biologically active and are not designed to be ingested as are pharmaceuticals, but they can and do often exhibit both traits).

(2) Slightly later, in 1976, the U.S. Congress made a different ethical choice with a law to protect the public from the large class of general chemicals; it chose *postmarket* laws to govern these creations that were in or would enter commerce (Cranor, 2017). This was contrary to the advice of the Council on

Environmental Quality (above), quite different from premarket testing laws that were already in existence, and, I will argue, unjust (Cranor, 2017).

Under postmarket laws there are no *routinely* required scientific tests of products to protect the public from the risks of toxicants; the postmarket laws neither demand independent scientific review nor expect from manufacturers reasonable assurances of a product's safety before it enters the market, thus exposing both the public and companies' workforces to that product whose safety has not been proven adequately. Few primordial preventions from toxic risks resulted. Ethically this law was not written to require the prudent and routine use of science to identify risks from toxicants until well after exposures, risks, and even harms have occurred. Instead, the law explicitly assumed that the U.S. Environmental Protection Agency could identify toxicants after being given only minimal information about products, and it implicitly seemed to assume quick risk assessments could identify risks from products in commerce before they materialized into harms. The assumption about risk assessments turned out to be a misguided hope.[2]

Postmarket laws ethically fail to adequately protect the public from risks or harms and fail to initiate improved health protections until some citizens have been clearly put at risk or actually harmed.

For *existing* chemicals TSCA grandfathered as "safe" an inventory of about 62,000 "general" substances manufactured or imported into the United States with few tested for toxicity. Any substances not on that inventory would be considered "new." These would have to be submitted to the EPA under premarket "notification" provisions (PMN). However, proposed new products were not required to undergo any routine toxicity testing and received only cursory agency review. If the EPA could discern toxic properties from the minimal PMN data, it could require toxicity tests—a quite time-consuming procedure (Cranor, 2017), but otherwise there was no requirement to conduct toxicity tests before products were approved for commercialization (U.S. General Accounting Office, 1994).

Thus, U.S. Congress's choices in writing this law permitted the public to be put at risk and perhaps harmed. Primordial protection from risks was not front and center in their concerns. With sufficient exposures and potencies either the general population or specific subpopulations might contract maladies from "approved" chemical products under this law.

Hairdresser Sandy Guest serves as one example (in addition to Brian Milward above). Ms. Guest used Brazilian Blowout, a hair-straightening product that was "loaded with formaldehyde" (Morris, 2015). She contracted leukemia because of high concentrations of formaldehyde and died of leukemia at age 55. This is heartrending because, beginning in 1981, as many as 17 different studies conducted over a period of 30 years revealed that formaldehyde could cause nasopharyngeal, sinonasal, and myeloid cancers, along with other disorders (Cranor, 2017). The U.S. public health institutions had evidence of formaldehyde's toxicity. However, even at this late date (2019), there are still no protections from formaldehyde for the general public, and Brazilian

Blowout appears still to contain formaldehyde. Two institutions—the company that made Brazilian Blowout and administrative institutions—failed her, causing her death and eliminating her full range of life's opportunities. A 30-year scientific record of formaldehyde's toxicity did not protect her.

Analogous problems arose from workplace and public exposures to Du-Pont's perfluorooctanoic acid (PFOA), also known as C8, the main ingredient in Teflon, Gore-Tex, stain-resistant fabrics, and flame-retardants, *inter alia*. Some DuPont employees in their prime of life developed testicular cancer along with cancers in the lymph nodes, while others contracted ulcerative colitis, which led to colorectal cancer (Lerner, 2015a). More broadly, individuals living near a DuPont plant and merely drinking tap water contaminated with C8, which was "pooped into the environment," contracted kidney and testicular cancers along with other C8-caused diseases (Steenland et al., 2013). Ohio courts compensated Carla Bartlett for kidney cancer ($1.6 million, in 2016) along with David Freeman ($5.6 million with punitive damages, in 2017) and Kenneth Vigneron, Sr. for testicular cancers ($12.5 million with punitive damages, in 2017; Cranor, 2017). DuPont settled with plaintiffs for $670.7 million to cover their damages and clean up their water supplies (Frisbee et al., 2009; Rinehart, 2017). The state of Minnesota independently recovered $850 million from 3M corporation to "remedy [C8] water-pollution problems of private well owners and cities" (Shaw, 2018).

3M and DuPont scientists developed C8, which they recognized to be toxic about 30 years ago but unethically failed to inform its own employees, the EPA (as legally required), and the public about its toxicity (Lerner, 2015a; Grandjean, 2018). In addition, EPA's sluggish action, likely the result of TSCA's provisions and the company's secrecy plus its resistance to regulation, led to workforce's and then the public's diseases. The company's unethical choices and the law's structure treated its employees and the general public unjustly—they were seriously harmed and many had their lifetime opportunities burdened, attenuated, or both.

However, while the tort law redressed some people with their disease treatments and perhaps prevented others from contracting diseases caused by C8, those settlements are likely limited. Often the tort law fails to fully restore a person to the condition he or she would have been in had he/she not contracted the disease. (2) Although the settlement likely will facilitate decontaminating water systems, somewhat correcting DuPont's disposal practices, it will probably do little overall to reduce C8 exposures. Because C8 is chemically quite stable—called the "forever chemical"—and has been incorporated into other products, for example, flame suppressants, it has now spread all over the world and contaminated 98% of U.S. citizens (Calafat et al., 2007; Slater, 2016).

These examples illustrate several important ethical issues. DuPont and before that 3M with awareness of the toxicity of C8 failed the public and its workforce, almost certainly violating the old TSCA by not reporting

C8's toxicity. This sluggish and illegal response unethically violated the FEOP and harmed identified and unidentified citizens who may never know what caused their diseases. The companies also illegally dumped C8 into the ground, rivers, and air (Lerner, 2015b). The EPA under a poorly protective postmarket law also ethically failed to protect the public, even as well as it might have under that flawed law.[3]

Health risks from products subject to postmarket regulation under old TSCA or pollutants under other postmarket laws, such as the Clean Water Act (CWA), Safe Drinking Water Act (SDWA), or the Clean Air Act (CAA), can only be reduced or eliminated if they have *already been legally identified as toxic* (and under CWA, SDWA, and CAA legally "listed" as toxic). Thus, such laws largely fail to protect the public and do not provide primordial disease prevention, hardly a health-protective ethical approach. Even worse, the last three laws are woefully out of date; C8 was not on CWA and SDWA lists of toxicants (Cranor, 2017; Mandel, 2019).

Ethical implications for research buttressing health protections

Legislative choices for post-exposure and post-risk laws that should, but do not, well-protect the public are only part of the story. There can also be ethical failures in how the tools of science are used for buttressing health protections. Public health agencies face particular scientific and political hurdles once companies' products are in commerce generating income for companies (Cranor, 2017, 2019). Products may pose public health threats yet may also have fierce defenders to resist their products' removal, reformulation, or reduction of risks because such actions will likely increase costs and reduce profit margins.

How much science is required to protect the public is a further ethical choice once products are in commerce. If too much science is required—"scientific overkill," or as I have characterized it, "ideal" or "doubt-free" science, this will greatly hamper public health protections, likely permitting more people to be harmed (Cranor, 2017). Moreover, if scientific studies are not conducted with integrity, generating "valid and accurate evidence on occupational and environmental hazards" (Collegium Ramazzini, 2018), this too will undermine or preclude sufficient protections of health.

Of course, needed scientific studies themselves can contribute to delays, because they can be slow, marching to their own drummers or perhaps to funeral dirges. In order to reveal diseases, epidemiological studies must allow for sufficient latency periods, from a few months up to 45 years. In studies conducted too soon after exposures, disease effects will often be missed. Rare diseases must be studied with sufficient samples to discover them (Cranor, 2017). Animal studies can take up to seven years to authorize, fund, conduct, and then interpret the results. The slower any studies document risks, if exposures are great enough, the more people will be harmed (Cranor, 2017; Neutra et al., 2018). Which studies are utilized to reveal toxic effects also involves important ethical decisions. Sometimes companies urge that only certain kinds of studies are appropriate for assessing the risks from their products, for example, epidemiological studies. However, these are notoriously insensitive in detecting disease risks.

Surprisingly, recently pesticide companies insisted that EPA utilize animal data and opposed human studies where people had been exposed to pesticides. The companies sought not only the studies, but also the underlying data, which researchers would not provide because of privacy concerns for their participants. For example, epidemiological studies have been utilized to identify neurological problems in children born to mothers who have had pesticide exposures in fieldwork. If researchers must reveal their "underlying data" about the people involved, this not only violates scientific commitments to privacy but likely also gives opponents material they can distort to undermine the science. Such data are requested to make studies more transparent, but the data seem more like "a caricature of how science really works", a caricature that "weaponizes transparency," according to David Michaels, former head of the U.S. Occupational Safety and Health Administration and an epidemiologist at George Washington School of Public Health (Hakim and Lipton, 2018). More importantly, it seems that the industry's underlying concern is that epidemiological studies came up with the wrong answers for products (Hakim and Lipton, 2018).

In contrast to demands that certain kinds of studies must be utilized or must not be utilized, administrative agencies (and the law more generally) must utilize appropriate combinations of epidemiological, experimental animal data, *in vitro*, and mechanistic evidence sufficient for identifying the toxicity and risks of products (Cranor, 2017) and not succumb to self-interested arguments for certain kinds of studies or for ideal or doubt-free science (next).

Company behavior exacerbates the inherent sluggishness of science. Most companies follow the tobacco industry in casting doubt on studies unfavorable to their products (Michaels, 2012) or urge that agencies utilize "ideal" scientific studies before reducing or removing risks (Cranor, 2017). Ideal studies might include several well-designed human epidemiological studies supported by good and valid animal data at exposure levels similar to human exposures, further corroborated by short-term tests and biological mechanisms that function similarly on analogous organs in humans and animals (Furst, 1990). And, all of these, companies urge, should be free of "doubt." Such proposals set very high scientific bars before agencies can act on toxicants and are likely proposed to paralyze health protections, continuing risks to the public. If agencies acquiesce in such strategies, the public will remain at risk and likely suffer more diseases. Typically, administrative agencies would be alert to such tactics, but legal requirements may force them to consider a range of unnecessary studies (Michaels, 2012).

Companies can adopt less scientifically honorable tactics in addition to those described two paragraphs above. These include

> hiring experts known to produce company-friendly outcomes, altering the outcome of study results, designing studies unlikely to find adverse effects that would require no change in protections, having lawyers "ghost-write" articles for scientific publication and then seeking scientists to sign on to the articles, and sometimes engaging in outright fraud as found by a court.
>
> (Cranor forthcoming, 2019b)

Some organizations like DuPont and 3M simply failed to follow the law and report toxicologically adverse effects (Grandjean, 2018). These approaches reveal greater or lesser ethical violations and scientific cheating, depending upon which tactic is used. A major commitment to primordially protect the public from the risks of harm and to better prevent their lifetime opportunities from being undermined was not in evidence.

How much science is needed and how quickly it can be employed to reduce or remove risks to protect the public is a further major ethical and institutional issue. Either using science deliberately to slow toxic determinations by clogging the regulatory agenda (Michaels, 2012) or demanding that the strictest science must be provided before reducing or removing risks will likely increase harm to individuals (Cranor, 2017).

Newly identified human susceptibility periods heightens ethical concerns for improved health protections for studies to identify subtle harms

The developmental origins of disease

A new and rapidly developing science—the developmental origins of disease—increases the ethical urgency to protect the public. This both calls attention to less emphasized persons needing protection and points to the need to develop scientific studies to better identify risks to children.

Children are among the most vulnerable humans exposed to toxicants (Grandjean et al., 2008; Cranor, 2011). How well do laws that have permitted harm to adults protect children? Three major disease catastrophes affecting human development early on signaled wider and more consequential problems with toxic exposures: *in utero* exposures to methylmercury, thalidomide, and diethylstilbestrol. Such exposures can harm one and begin to truncate opportunities early in life.

Methylmercury, dumped into Minamata Bay in Japan, was absorbed by fish, which people, including pregnant women, ingested thus exposing children to methylmercury *in utero* (1950s). Some children were born with cerebral palsy, but many also had, *inter alia,* neurological problems, auditory disturbance, limb deformities, and poor muscle control. Some mothers miscarried or their children were stillborn (Masazumi, 1995; McCurry, 2006).

In the 1960s, women were encouraged to use the sedative Thalidomide during the first trimester of pregnancy, the period when they suffer morning sickness and fail to sleep well. This *in utero* pharmaceutical exposure caused newborns to have shortened or displaced limbs, along with spinal malformations, kidney abnormalities, autism, and some other learning disabilities, *inter alia*. About 5,000–7,000 children worldwide were affected, but only about 40 in the United States (Cranor, 2011). Another 7,000–8,000 children worldwide naturally aborted or were stillborn (Schardein and Macina, 2007).

Finally, in the 1950s–1960s, physicians mistakenly believed that pregnant women with a history of miscarriages should take the synthetic estrogen diethylstilbestrol (DES) to help prevent miscarriages. Female children born to women who took DES were 40 times more likely to contract vaginal/cervical cancer after a 20-year latency period than women not so exposed (U.S. National Institutes of Health). The DES "daughters" were also at increased and earlier risk of breast cancer than non-exposed adults because of DES exposure (U.S. National Institutes of Health). They may also convey risks to their offspring (U.S. National Institutes of Health).

Research into the "developmental origins of disease" (Grandjean et al., 2008) has revealed toxic harm caused early in life necessitated a more radical and long-needed ethical reassessment to protect children *in utero* and in early life (Cranor, 2011). Children's vulnerability to toxicants upped the public health stakes and increased the need for more in-depth and exhaustive scientific studies conducted with integrity in order to identify early-life harms. Since postmarket laws are inadequate to protect adults from toxicants, children with long lives ahead of them are at greater risk (Cranor, 2011, 2017).

Chronic diseases in humans can originate from environmental insults during development and beyond—from embryos to fetuses to infants to teenagers (Cao, 2016) even to later life stages (Heindel, 2018). Young humans' organs and cells are more easily damaged. They have greater exposures per body weight via umbilical cord blood, breast milk, and higher rates of inhalation and respiration after birth. They have lesser defenses against toxic invasions, and they have a longer lifespan for diseases to develop if exposures initiate them. Moreover, since toxic effects on the brain, immune system, and (likely) reproductive systems are irreversible—developing children have just one chance "to get right" the healthy development of these organ systems (Grandjean, 2008; Cranor, 2017).

Toxic contamination is widespread. Up to 300-plus manmade toxicants contaminate citizens (U.S. Department of Health and Human Services, 2019). Pregnant women can harbor 43-plus toxicants that contaminate developing children *in utero* (Woodruff et al., 2011): There is "no placental barrier per se: the vast majority of chemicals given to pregnant animal (or woman) reach the fetus in significant concentrations soon after administration" (Schardein,

2000). Plastic nanoparticles have joined the invasions (Wick et al., 2010). Newborns enter the world harboring toxicants (Fimrite, 2009).

Susceptibility genes add to the vulnerability of some people to some toxicants—polycyclic aromatic hydrocarbons (by-products of combustion; Perera et al., 1999), organophosphate pesticides (Furlong et al., 2006), and methylmercury (Julez et al., 2013). Moreover, most childhood cancers begin in the womb, for example, acute lymphoblastic (ALL) and acute myeloid childhood leukemias (AML) (Ross, 1999; Greaves and Wiemels, 2003; McHale and Smith, 2004).

In utero and even early-life exposures are especially risky because children are ultrasensitive to tiny doses of toxicants; for example, mutagenic carcinogens have no threshold for toxicity (Eastmond, 2012), lead exposures have no identified safe level (Lanphear, 2000; Bellinger and Needleman, 2003; Canfield, 2003), and a single Thalidomide pill can cause malformations (Claudio, 2000). Ethically public health officials should understand that even substances that act via thresholds in individuals can produce linear effects in large heterogeneous populations, in effect having no lowest threshold for the most susceptible individuals, including children (Lutz, 1990, 2001).

Animal studies reveal that *in utero* exposures to toxicants during reproductive organ development can cause transgenerational reproductive harm along with some cancers and other maladies in males and females alike (Manikkam et al., 2012; Nilsson et al., 2012).

Many of these adverse effects are subtle and often take time to identify—especially the adverse neurological effects in children. Some can take even longer when there are substantial delays between exposures and diseases or dysfunctions. It is important that such studies be conducted with scientific integrity and not be undermined out of self-interested commercial concerns as seems to be occurring with industry protests against the use of human epidemiological studies.

Moreover, children are not merely exposed and at risk; they have been *harmed* and had their opportunities truncated. The estimated *annual* costs of pediatric diseases of environmental origin include the following: lead ($50.9 billion), methylmercury ($5.1 billion), asthma ($2.2 billion), intellectual disability ($5.4 billion), autism ($7.9 billion), attention deficit hyperactivity disorder (ADHD; $5.0 billion), and childhood cancer ($95 million), with a best total estimate of these diseases of $76.6 billion (Transande and Liu, 2011).

Workplace exposures can also put children at risk

Another hidden and quite subtle, but not surprising, source of toxic exposures for children occurs from occupational settings, revealing further consequences of poor protections for workers. Of course, women who are exposed to and carry toxicants in their bodies will convey them to developing fetuses. However, fathers contaminated with Paxil, anesthetic gases, morphine, lead, mercury, pesticides, solvents, dyes, and paints can also be a reason for miscarriages along with prenatal or neonatal problems in their children (An-thes, 2010). Moreover, because protections for workers tend to be so poor, some say employees are "callously" unprotected (Morris, 2015a), this creates largely hidden disease risks for their children. For instance, Yvette Flores worked in an electronics plant and her "body was a 'toxic warehouse before [her son] Mark was conceived'" (Morris, 2015a). Mark was born with "ex-tensive cognitive impairment" caused by *in utero* lead exposures. Now 36, he has no ordinary opportunities; he cannot care for himself the rest of his life. Yvette's place of work, Spectra-Physics, along with the Occupational Safety and Health Administration, failed both Yvette and her son Mark (Cra-nor, 2017). While occupational exposures can put both adults and developing children at risk, workplaces poorly protect employees. Increased health pro-tections are especially needed in this area (Finkel, 2019).

Later-life periods of vulnerability

Puberty constitutes another period of vulnerability. Young women with DDT exposures around the time of puberty contracted breast cancer 20 years later at rates five times higher than adult women with comparable exposures (Cohn et al., 2007). Women born to mothers with substantial *in utero* expo-sures to DDT contract breast cancer at rates four times higher than women not exposed *in utero* (Cohn et al., 2007, 2015). Radiation "increases breast cancer risk most strongly when exposures occur early in life" (Miller et al., 2002; Ronckers et al., 2004).

The developmental basis of disease and our permeability to toxicants places in even starker relief both the ethical shortcomings of postmarket laws (along with the urgency to improve them) and the need to conduct scientific re-search with integrity to identify the often-subtle effects. We cannot prevent human permeability or developmental vulnerability to toxicants, but we can better preclude—primordially—toxic risks.

In addition, humans, especially, but not only, women, go through sev-eral stages of susceptibility to diseases. Greater susceptibility typically occurs "during fetal life, early childhood, adolescence, and early reproductive life, particularly before the first full-term pregnancy" (Heindel, 2018). Mam-malian models strongly show notable periods of vulnerability to toxicant-triggered diseases in different life stages (Heindel, 2018).

Timeline of Vulnerable Life Stages in a Person and Her Offspring.

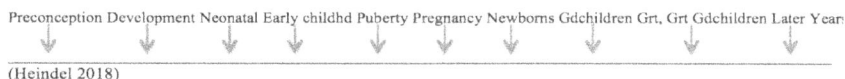

Preconception Development Neonatal Early childhd Puberty Pregnancy Newborns Gdchildren Grt, Grt Gdchildren Later Years

(Heindel 2018)

Thus, some of us may be exposed prenatally, but even if we avoid diseases at that time, we may not escape toxicant-induced maladies. Potential early-life exposures may be augmented, creating risks later in life. Thus, considering this issue as part of community justice, it is important ethically to understand the different vulnerability periods and seek to ensure primordial protection from the risks if we care about the wider public's health. These newly identified periods of vulnerability open up additional areas of research and require scientists to specifically look for adverse effects from exposures in later life and to consider the effects of cumulative and additive exposures that could occur during other susceptibility periods.

Researchers will need to develop research strategies to determine whether products cause (possibly subtle) adverse effects at different life stages, in order to support legal protections. If adverse effects are revealed at multiple life stages, legal strategies to protect the public should be quickly adopted (Cranor, 2017; Heindel, 2018).

Learning from physicians we should aspire to "primordial prevention" of harm—preventing *risk factors* from toxicants as best we can for many different vulnerability stages of life. Just as the best approach to avoiding lung cancer from smoking is to never smoke, community health-protective institutions with the best scientific tools available ethically should aspire to identify and prevent (or remove) risks from toxic substances that could affect people at many different life stages.

Of course, this is a tall order, given how postmarket laws have permitted toxic products into the public sphere, while substantially burdening and frustrating their removal. Remnants of some of those toxicants will remain for some time.

A legal improvement, but ethical issues reappear

The discussion has focused on shortcomings of postmarket laws and some of the ethical issues they pose, because they have long been part of the U.S. legal system, are likely part of numerous other legal systems, and leave a legacy of thousands of untested products in commerce. Fortunately, the U.S. Congress finally updated and improved a law for general chemical products, the Frank R. Lautenberg Chemical Safety for the 21st Century Act (U.S. EPA, 2016; Cranor, 2017). This law requires the EPA to affirm a substance is appropriately "safe"—somewhat resembling premarket review provisions—and endorses the protection of susceptible and highly exposed subpopulations, including infants, pregnant women, children, and workers. It also has some enforceable timelines for reviewing the toxicity of existing products in commerce (US EPA, 2016).

This law does seem to represent an ethical improvement on and does seem to be somewhat more coherent, precise, and broader in its stipulations concerning ethics than the old TSCA. Even so, substantial ethical shortcomings can reappear in its implementation. In the United States, a decidedly antireg ulatory Presidential administration is creating the policies to implement the Lautenberg Act. Administrators seem to be failing in their duties to protect the public (Eilpern and Dennis, 2017).

Distortion of the Lautenberg Act would occur if the EPA asserted as "safe" new products with little or no toxicity testing and then asymmetrically insisted on quite detailed and certain evidence of health risks before reducing or removing them. While there has been a limited track record, in 2017 the EPA administrator, a well-known antiregulatory lawyer, immediately approved 600 new substances for commerce, probably with limited evidence (Chow, 2017; Eilpern and Dennis, 2017; Henry, 2017). Were any toxicants identified and precluded from commerce with such a quick review? Were toxicants permitted in? It seems unlikely they were well reviewed for toxicity, but it could take decades to reveal any shortcomings, leaving the public as experimental subjects in the meantime.

An additional distortion of science is that the U.S. EPA in the Trump administration was pushing to adopt the restrictions on scientific studies urged by industry discussed above concerning pesticides (Hakim and Lipton, 2018).

Data are limited in showing how the agency will remove health risks from products already in commerce. Will this continue to be plagued by delays, demands for doubt-free science, and extensive industry resistance? However, reviewing even as few as 30,000 active substances in commerce will be a decades-long, if not a centuries-long, task, likely leaving some citizens at risk (Cranor, 2017).

The ethical (or non-ethical) approaches to implementing Lautenberg Act are far from reassuring and probably will not serve the public well. While early indications bode ill for the public, that history still needs to be written, but it will be difficult to determine the causes of diseases because of the difficulties in tracing causal paths from the past.

Some summary remarks

First, serious chronic diseases, the disruptions they cause, toxicants' contributions to them, the manner in which postmarket laws function, the presence of numerous chemical products in the environment, the vulnerability of developing children, and humans' general vulnerability to toxicants during a lifetime, all raise substantial ethical issues for how research is conducted, how legislation is written, and how it is administered to protect the public's health, a preeminent justice concern. Together these concerns greatly strengthen the need for premarket toxicity testing of industrial chemicals supported by scientific studies conducted with integrity, somewhat analogous to the testing of pharmaceuticals and pesticides in the United States and to physicians' recommended primordial prevention of disease risks. Justice also gives top priority to research and legal strategies to prevent diseases and dysfunctions that cause harm and/or opportunity-truncating effects compared with good health over a lifetime (Fries, 1980; Daniels, 1981; Cranor, 2017).

These considerations also accentuate substantial cognitive dissonance in ethical choices that arise between different institutions. To see this, conduct the following *Gedankenspiel* (thought play).

Suppose you are a woman, follow your doctor's advice based on previous scientific studies, take care of your health, exercise to increase the reserves of your organ systems, and are a "compliant patient" in taking any prescribed pharmaceuticals. However, suppose that you, like Yvette Flores, work in an electronics factory with substantial exposures to lead, other heavy metals, and some additional toxicants that have previously been revealed in good scientific studies. Suppose these in turn cause a serious neurological condition for you and contaminate your developing child *in utero*.

Or imagine the same scenario, but not including extensive exposure to lead. Now suppose you merely drink tap water contaminated with C8. You might begin to have symptoms of ulcerative colitis, thyroid disease, or even kidney cancer. This from merely drinking local tap water system, as did citizens of Ohio and West Virginia.

The point? Some institutions and health-protective choices aspire to primordial prevention of health risks, foster good health, and contribute to a long and flourishing life with wide opportunities. However, for public health institutions governing workplace (where we spend about one-third of our lives) and general laws permitting environmental exposures there will need to be health protections supported by scientific studies conducted with integrity so that your, your child's, and others' health are not undermined. That is, failures of current or quite recent environmental health laws, unethical research that distorts health-protective efforts, and company behavior along the way simultaneously poorly protect your health, undermine and undo the goals of other health institutions, and frustrate gains you can personally achieve by having good health habits. Some actors in countries work overtime to frustrate science conducted with integrity that supports either the need for additional administrative protections or new legislation to better protect the public.

We live with this cognitive and ethical dissonance in today's world. Because of the importance of good health to each of our lives, opportunities, and longevity should we not have a more unified approach to scientific research that better supports people's health and any needed legal modifications to accomplish this aim? Should we not insist that public health institutions converge in their protections for our health supported by research conducted with integrity that serves these aims?

Primordial protection of patients from the health risks of prescription drugs and pesticides seems quite sensible and suggests similar approaches to general chemicals. However, some may resist the approach suggested above. Will there be valuable commercial substances with some low level of risks that are critical to the economy; should these be permitted? (Table 4.2).

Some uses of lead, especially in electronics, are likely examples. Lead is quite toxic with no known lowest safe level (Wigle and Lanphear, 2005), but it may still be needed in our electronic world. Even if it is, primordial prevention still seems appropriate. The production and recycling of products incorporating lead should be organized to protect employees from neurological

Table 4.2 Tiered prevention institutional strategies

Legal-institutional responses	**Prevent risks that can lead to diseases—** screen human-created chemicals for toxicity with premarket testing and scientific review laws, for example, FDCA, new TSCA, pesticide laws.	**Expeditiously reduce exposures posing risks** once identified—use **postmarket risk reduction** or postmarket correctives under premarket laws.	**Reduce exposures** but provide means of treatment with torts—use **postmarket regulatory actions** plus tort actions for compensation.	**Reduce morbid states as best one can** when they are caused by others' toxicants —use the tort (personal injury) law.

Reconstructed from Fries et al. (2011).

disorders. This has not always been the case, even for children living near lead reclamation facilities (Frankel, 2011; Walter, 2012).

Chlorinating drinking water presents a similar example, but shows a health benefit-versus-health risk tradeoff. Chlorination treatments prevent risks from some diseases in drinking water. The chlorine interacts with organic matter to create trihalomethane, a weak carcinogen. Importantly, a risk assessment supports this use of chlorine—potentially substantial health risks are prevented by chlorination but with low levels of carcinogenic risks. This health-health assessment is certainly worth taking (Cranor, 2011). However, if there were less risky methods of purifying drinking water at a comparable or even somewhat higher cost, primordial prevention of the risks of disease would argue for adopting those.

When we face such tradeoffs we should aspire primordially to protect the public's health. We can have more convergent health care and public health protections if we ethically choose to do so in a variety of circumstances. This will take changes in choices and behavior in creating and administering more health-protective legal institutions supported by ethnically sound scientific studies in a unified medico-legal approach to good health.

Notes

1 Three precepts of justice supported by FEOP guide the prevention and treatment of disease by basic institutions. These require that community institutions
   i) prevent diseases in the first place, including environmental health and work-place diseases;
   ii) provide adequate and timely treatment for those who contract diseases; and

    iii) maintain people as close as possible to normal biological functioning over a
        complete lifetime (Daniels, 1981; Cranor, 2017).
  2 Premarket laws for pharmaceuticals and pesticides govern only about 10–20% of
      the chemical creations by manufacturers, while the 1976 Toxic Substances Con-
      trol Act (call it "old" TSCA) largely governs about 80–90% of the general chem-
      ical creations, excluding small numbers of prescription drugs, pesticides, tobacco
      products, nuclear material, foods, new food additives, chemical mixtures, and
      cosmetic ingredients (U.S. General Accounting Office, 1994).
  3 The Occupational Safety and Health Act, which governs workplace exposures,
      is also a postmarket law that is poorly administered, providing few protections in
      the workplace; space does not permit its discussion here (Finkel, 2019; Cranor,
      forthcoming, 2019a).

References

American College of Obstetricians and Gynecologists Committee on Health Care for Underserved Women, American Society for Reproductive Medicine Practice Committee, with the assistance of the University of California at San Francisco (UCSF) Program on Reproductive Health and the Environment. 'Committee Opinion: Exposure to Toxic Environmental Agents.' Committee Opinion 575, October 2013.

Anthes E. (2010) 'The Bad Daddy Factor Drinking, Smoking, Taking Prescription Meds or Failing to Eat a Balanced Diet Can Influence the Health of Men's Future Children', Pacific Standard. www.psmag.com/books-and-culture/thebad-daddy-factor-25764 [Accessed June 2015].

Bellinger B. and Needleman H. L. (2003) 'Intellectual impairment and blood lead levels', New England Journal of Medicine 349, 500–502.

Canfield, R. L., Kreher, D.A., Cornwell, C and Henderson Jr., C.R. (2003) 'Low-Level Lead Exposure, Executive Functioning, and Learning in Early Childhood', *Child Neuropsychology* 9.1: 35–53.

Calafat A., Wong L-Y., Kuklenyik Z., Reidy J.A., and Needham L.L. (2007) Poly-fluoroalkyl Chemicals in the U.S. Population: Data from the National Health and Nutrition Examination Survey (NHANES) 2003–2004 and Comparisons with NHANES 1999–2000, *Environ Health Perspectives*, 115:1596–1602

Cao J., MS, Xu X., Hylkema M.N., (2016) 'Early-life Exposure to Widespread Environmental Toxicants and Health Risk: A Focus on the Immune and Respiratory Systems', *Annals of Global 82 119–131*. Available at http://dx.doi.org/10.10 6/j.aogh.2016.01.023.

Chow L. (2017) 'Industry Friendly' EPA Completes Review of 600 New Chemicals, *EcoWatch*. Available at https://www.ecowatch.com/epa-approves-chemicals-2470558970.html.

Claudio L., Kwa W. C., Russell A. L., et al. (2000) 'Testing Methods for Developmental Neurotoxicity of Environmental Chemicals', *Toxicology and Applied Pharmacology*, 164, 1–14.

Cohn B. A., Wolff M.S., Cirillo P. M., and Sholtz, R. I. et al., (2007) 'DDT and Breast Cancer in Young Women: New Data on the Significance of Age at Exposure', *Environmental Health Perspectives*, 115.10: 1406–14,

Cohn B. A., LaMerrill, M., Krigbaum, N. Y., et al. (2015) 'DDT Exposure in Utero and Breast Cancer', *Journal of Endocrinology & Metabolism* 100.8 (2015): 2865–72.

Cranor C. F. (2011) *Legally Poisoned: How the Law Puts Us at Risk from Toxicants.* Cambridge, MA: Harvard University Press.

Cranor C. F. (2018) 'The Interaction of Science and Law in Protecting the Public's Health', European Journal of Oncology, 23(3): 165–175, 2018

Cranor C.F. (forthcoming 2019a) 'Justice and Ethical Duties in Occupational Safety and Medicine'. *Current Occupational and Environmental Medicine, 6th Edition*, Ed. Joe LaDou and Robert Harrison, Lange Medical Books, McGraw-Hill

Cranor C. F. (2016) *Toxic Torts: Science, Law and the Possibility of Justice. 2d Edition.* New York and Cambridge, UK; Cambridge University Press.

Cranor C. F. (2017) *Tragic Failures: How and Why We Are Harmed by Toxic Substances.* New York and Oxford: Oxford University Press.

Daniels N: Health-Care Needs and Distributive Justice. (1981) *Philosophy and Public Affairs*, 10:2, 146–179.

Eastmond D. A. (2012) 'Personal Communication' University of California, Environmental Toxicology Program.

Eilpern J. and Dennis B. (2017) Scott Pruitt, Outspoken and Forceful, Moves to the Center of Power within the Trump Administration, *Washingon Post*, June 2, 2017. Available at https://www.washingtonpost.com/politics/scott-pruittoutspoken-and-forceful-moves-to-the-center-of-power-within-the-trumpadministration/2017/06/02/a1b4d298-46fa-11e7-a196-a1bb629f64cb_story.html?utm_term=.5750e5dce6b8.

Frankel T.C.(2011) $320 million verdict in lead smelter case sends clear message, *Saint Louis Today*, Metro Division July 30, 2011. Available at http://www.stltoday.com/news/local/metro/million-verdict-in-lead-smeltercase-sends-clear-message/article_12f7e0ba-29ab-5894-8067-9a45ad255cfa.html.

Fimrite P. (2009) 'Study: Chemicals, Pollutants Found in Newborns', *SFGate*, Available at http:// www.sfgate.com/ health/ article/ Study-Chemicals-pollutants-found-in-newborns-3207709.php.

Finkel A. M. (2019) Hearing on "Mismanaging Chemical Risks: EPA's Failure to Protect Workers," Testimony of Adam M. Finkel, Sc.D., CIH, Clinical Professor of Environmental Health Sciences, University of Michigan School of Public Health, Before the U.S. House of Representatives Committee on Energy and Commerce Environment and Climate Change Subcommittee

Fries J. F. (1980) 'Aging, Natural Death, and the Compression of Morbidity', *New England Journal of Medicine*, 80(3), 130–135.

Fries J. F. Bruce B., and Chakravarty E. (2011) 'Compression of Morbidity 1980–2011: A Focused Review of Paradigms and Progress', *Journal of Aging Research*, 2011, Article ID 261702.

Frisbee B., Books, A.P., Maher A., et al. (2009) 'The C8 Health Project: Design, Methods, and Participants', *Environmental Health Perspectives*, 117(12), 1873–1882.

Furlong C.E., Holland N., Richter R.J., Bradman A, Ho A., and Eskenazi B. (2006) "PON1 Status of Farmworker Mothers and Children as a Predictor of Organophosphate Sensitivity," *Pharmacogenetics and Genomics* 16, 183–190.

Furst A. (1990) "Yes, but is it a human carcinogen?" *Journal of the American College of Toxicology*, 9, (1), 1–18.

Grandjean P. (2018) Delayed Discovery, Dissemination, and Decisions on Intervention in Environmental Health: A Case Study on Immunotoxicity of Perfluorinated Alkylate Substances, Environmental Health, 17:62–68. Available at https://doi.org/10.1186/s12940-018-0405-y.

Grandjean P., Bellinger D., Bergman A., Cordier S., Davey-Smith G., Eskenazi B., Gee D., et al. (2007) "The Faroes Statement: Human Health Effects of Developmental Exposure to Chemicals in Our Environment', *Basic & Clinical Pharmacology & Toxicology* 102.2 (2008): 73–5.

Greaves M. F., Wiemels J. (2003) "Origins of Chromosome Translocations in childhood Leukeaemia, *Nature Reviews Cancer* 3.9: 639–49.

Hakim D and Lipton E (2018) Pesticide Studies Won E.P.A.'s Trust, Until Trump's Team Scorned 'Secret Science.' New York Times, August 24, 2018.

Heindel, J. (2018) 'The developmental basis of disease: Update on environmental exposures and animal models', *Basic and Clinical Pharmacology and Toxicology*, 1–9, located at DOI: 10.1111/bcpt.13118.

Henry D. (2017) *The Hill*, 08/07/17. Available at https://thehill.com/policy/energyenvironment/345650-epa-completes-review-of-chemical-approval-backlog.

Julvez J., Smith G.D., Golding J., Ring S., St. Pourcain B., Gonzalez J.R., and Grandjean P. (2013) 'Prenatal Methylmercury Exposure and Genetic Predisposition to Cognitive Deficit at Age 8 Years', *Epidemiology*, 24.5, 643–50.

Lerner, S. (2015a) 'The Teflon Toxin: DuPont and the Chemistry of Deception', *The Intercept*, August, 11, 2015a. Available at https://theintercept.com/2015/08/11/dupont-chemistry-deception/.

Lerner, S. (2015 b) "The Teflon Toxin: The Case against DuPont," *The Intercept*, Available at https://theintercept.com/2015/08/17/teflon-toxin-case-againstdupont/.

Lombardi K. (2014) 'Benzene and Worker Cancers: An American Tragedy', Center for Public Integrity, available at http://www.publicintegrity.org/2014/12/04/16320/benzene-and-workercancers-american-tragedy.

Lutz, W.K. (1990) 'Dose-Response Relationship and Low-Dose Extrapolation in Carcinogenesis, *Carcinogenesis*, 11 (8), 1243–1247.

Lutz, W. K. (2001) 'Susceptibility differences in chemical carcinogenesis linearize the dose–response relationship: threshold doses can be defined only for individuals,' *Mutation Research*, 482, 71–76

Mancini J. (2017) 'DuPont Reaches C8 Settlement Agreement for $670M', *The Parkersburg News and Sentinel*. Available at http://www.newsandsentinel.com/news/local-news/2017/02/dupont-reachesc8-settlement-agreement-for-670m/.

Mandel, K. (2019) 'EPA's "Secret Science" Proposal Being Used by Big Oil Undermine Clean Water Rules: Fossil Fuel Trade Groups Don't Want the EPA to Update a 1970s-era List of Polluting Petroleum Chemicals, located at https://vidmid.com/news/epa-s-secret-science-proposal-being-used-by-big-oilto-undermine-clean-water-rules?uid=111722.

Manikkam M., Guerrero-Bosagna C., Tracey R., Haque M., and Skinner M.K.(2012) 'Transgenerational Actions of Environmental Compounds on Reproductive Disease and Identification of Epigenetic Biomarkers of Ancestral Exposures', *PLoS ONE* 7.2, e31901

Masazumi H. (1995) 'Minamata Disease: Methylmercury Poisoning in Japan Caused by Environmental Pollution', *Critical Reviews in Toxicology*," 25(1), 1–24,

McCurry J. (2006) 'Japan Remembers Minamata', *Lancet* 367.9505, 99–100.

MedicineNet; Medical Definition of Chronic disease, located at http://www.medicinenet.com/script/main/art.asp?articlekey=33490

Michaels D. (2012) *Doubt Is Their Product: How Industry's Assault on Science Threatens Your Health*. New York, NY: Oxford University Press.

Miller M. D., Marty M. A., Arcus A., Brown J., Morry D., and Sandy M. (2002) 'Differences between Children and Adults: Implications for Risk Assessment at California EPA', *International Journal of Toxicology* 21.5: 403–18.

Milward v. Acuity Specialty Products, Inc., 369 F 3d 11 (2011).

Morris J. (2016a) "About 'Science for Sale': The Danger of Tainted Science." *Center for Public Integrity*, February 18, 2016b. Available at http://www.publicintegrity.org/2016/02/08/19291/about-science-sale.

Morris J. (2015a) 'A Toxic Legacy', Toxic substances in electronics manufacturing: The U.S. does tragically little to protect workers from them. Money Box: Commentary about Business and Finance, Available at http://www.slate.com/articles/business/moneybox/2015/07/toxic_substancesin_electronics_manufacturing_the_u_s_does_tragically_little.html

Morris J. (2016b) 'Ford Spent $40 Million to Reshape Asbestos Science', Center for Public Integrity, Available at http://www.publicintegrity.org/2016/02/16/19297/ford-spent-40-millionreshape-asbestos-science.

Morris J. (2015b) "She Loved Making People Feel Great: Sandy Guest, 55, Hairdresser," Center for Public Integrity, Available at https://www.publicintegrity.org/2015/06/29/17533/she-loved-making-peoplefeel-great.

Myron A. Melman (1992) "Dangerous and Cancer-Causing Properties of Products and Chemicals in the Oil Refining and Petrochemical Industry," *Environmental Research* 59, 238–249.

National Research Council (NRC). (2014) *Review of Formaldehyde Assessment in the National Toxicology Program 12th Report on Carcinogens*. Washington, DC: National Academies Press.

Neutra R.R., Cranor C.F., Gee D. (2019) 'The Use and Abuse of Bradford Hill in U.S. Toxic Tort Litigation', Jurimetrics J, 58, 127–162.

Nilsson, E., Larsen, G. Manikkam, M., Guerrrero-Bosgna, C. Savenkova, M.I., and Skinner, M.K. 2012. "Environmentally Induced Epigenetic Transgenerational Inheritance of Ovarian Disease." PLoS One 7.5: e36129.

Perera F. P., Jedrychowski W., Rauh V., and Whyatt R.M. (1999) "Molecular Epidemiologic Research on the Effects of Environmental Pollutants on the Fetus', *Environmental Health Perspectives*, 107.S3, 451–60.

Rawls J. (1999) *A Theory of Justice, Revised Edition*, Cambridge, MA, Harvard University Press.

Rinehart E. (2017) "DuPont to pay $670 million to settle C8 lawsuits," *The Columbus Dispatch*, Feb 13, 2017. Available at http://www.dispatch.com/news/20170213/dupont-to-pay-670-million-to-settlec8-lawsuits.

Ronckers CM, Erdmann CA and Land CE (2004) 'Radiation and breast cancer: a review of current evidence', *Breast Cancer Research* 7 (1), 21–32.

Ross, JA *et al.*, (1999) Epidemiology of Childhood Leukemia, with a Focus on Infants, *Epidemiological Reviews*: 16(2): 243–272.

Shaw, B. (2018) 'Minnesota, 3M reach settlement ending $5 billion lawsuit'. Available at https://www.twincities.com/2018/02/20/minnesota-3m-reachsettlement-ending-5-billion-lawsuit/.

Shulevitz J. (2012) "Why Fathers Really Matter." *New York Time*. Available at http://nyti.ms/QavdtZ.

Schardein J. L. (2000) *Chemically Induced Birth Defects*. 3rd ed., rev. and expanded. New York: Marcel Dekker.

Schardein J. L. and Macina O.T. (2007) *Human Developmental Toxicants: Aspects of Toxicology and Chemistry*. Boca Raton, FL, Taylor & Francis.

Schierow L. (2007) *The Toxic Substances Control Act (TSCA): Implementation and New Challenges*. CRS Report for Congress RL34118. Washington, DC: Congressional Research Service, Library of Congress.

Slater J. (2016) 'Harvard Study on C8 Contamination', Available at https://slaterzurz. com/harvard-study-c8-contamination/.

McHale C.M., Smith M.T. (2004) 'Prenatal Origin of Chromosomal Translocations in Acute Childhood Leukemia: Implications and Future Directions', *American Journal of Hematology*, 75, 25425–25427.

Steenland, Kyle, Liping Zhao, Andrea Winquist, and Christine Parks (2013) "Ulcerative Colitis and Perfluorooctanoic Acid (PFOA) in a Highly Exposed Population of Community Residents and Workers in the Mid-Ohio Valley." *Environmental Health Perspectives* 121.8: 900–5. Available at http://dx.doi. org/10.1289/ehp.1206449.

Trasande L, Liu Y. (2011) 'Reducing the Staggering Costs of Environmental Disease in Children, Estimated at $76.6 Billion in 2008', *Health Affairs*. 30, 1–8.

US Congress, Office of Technology Assessment. *Identifying and Regulating Carcinogens.* Washington, DC: US Government Printing Office, 1987.

US Council on Environmental Quality (1971) *Toxic Substances*, Washington, DC: US Government Printing Office.

US Department of Health and Human Services, Centers for Disease Control and Prevention (2009) Fourth National Report on Human Exposure to Environmental Chemicals. Available at https://www.cdc.gov/exposurereport/pdf/FourthReport_ ExecutiveSummary.pdf.

US Department of Health and Human Services, Centers for Disease Control and Prevention (2019) 'National Report on Human Exposure to Environmental Chemicals (update of Fourth annual Report). Available at https://www.cdc.gov/ exposurereport/index.html.

US EPA. (2016) "Assessing and Managing Chemicals under TSCA: Highlights of Key Provisions in the Frank R. Lautenberg Chemical Safety for the 21st Century Act." Available at https://www.epa.gov/assessing-and-managingchemicals-under-tsca/ highlights-key-provisions-frank-r-lautenberg-chemical.

US Government Accountability Office (GAO), *Chemical Assessments: Low Productivity and New Interagency Review Process Limit the Usefulness and Credibility of EPA's Integrated Risk Information System*, GAO-08-440. Washington, DC: US Government Accountability Office, March 2008.

US National Institutes of Health, National Cancer Institute, "Diethystilbestrol (DES) and Cancer," available at http://www.cancer.gov/cancertopics/causesprevention/ risk/hormones/des-fact-sheet.

Walter D. (2012) Missouri Lawyers of the Year win $358M toxic tort case, *Missouri Lawyers Weekly*, January 27, 2012. Available at http://molawyersmedia.com/ 2012/01/27/video-missouri-lawyers-of-the-year/.

Wick, Peter, Antoine Malek, Pius Manser, Danielle Meili, Xenia Maeder-Althaus, Liliane Diener, Pierre-Andre Diener, Andreas Zisch, Harald F. Krug, and Ursula von Mandach. "Barrier Capacity of Human Placenta for Nanosized Materials." *Environmental Health Perspectives* 118.3 (2010): 432–6.

Wigle, D.T., Lanphear B.P. (2005) 'Human Health Risks from Low-Level Environmental Exposures: No Apparent Safety Thresholds', *PLoS Medicine*, 2.12, e350.

Woodruff T. J., Zota A.R, and Schwartz J.M. (2011) 'Environmental Chemicals in Pregnant Women In the United States: NHANES 2003–2004', *Environmental Health Perspectives*, 119.6, 878–885.

5 Connecting the dots

Toxicological decision-making and communication in the 21st century

Steven G. Gilbert

> It is not the <u>truth</u> that makes you free. It is your possession of the power to discover the truth. Our dilemma is that we do not know how to provide that power.
>
> Richard Lewontin (New York Review of Books, January 7, 1997)

Introduction

Scientists, public health professionals, and policymakers are in the business of exploring, developing, and communicating facts, and making decisions and even policies. But often the greatest challenge for those who use this information is not in identifying the scientific facts, but rather in effectively communicating and acting on those facts in a way that puts information in context with the past and within the expectations of a civil society. This chapter describes a new strategy: "Connecting the Dots" (CtD), which takes an identified problem and develops a framework of scientific facts, history, and ethics that supports and guides suggested action(s) to address the problem (Figure 5.1). Putting scientific facts within this framework provides concerned citizens, communities, organizations, scientists, and policymakers with the tools to understand and use information. The goal is to provide a tool to help organize information to address a problem and persuade policymakers or others to make changes and take action. Ultimately, this can enhance everyone's ability to carefully explore an approach to a problem, concisely communicate that information, and ultimately direct and take action.

Problem identification

Advances in science and technology have produced not only enormous benefits but have also created undesirable hazardous effects that impact human and environmental health. Despite the increased scientific data and understanding, decision-making has become more difficult and complex. It is also important to consider the ethical, historical, legal, economic, and social issues that confront toxicologists, public health professional, and decision-makers.

DOI: 10.4324/9780429318436-8

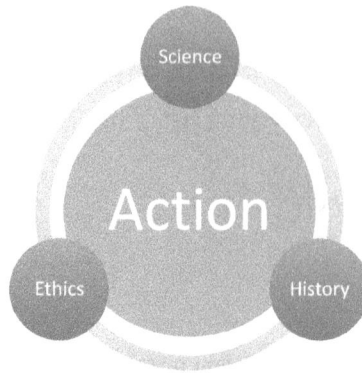

Figure 5.1 Connecting the dots (CtD).

It is with these considerations in mind that a method to connecting the facts of science, historical analysis, and ethics together to promote or discourage a specific action needs to be developed. Developing a CtD story is a multistep effort starting with identifying the problem; doing research on the science, history, and related ethical principles; then developing an action designed to address the identified problem; and finally crafting it all into a succinct story. The CtD is a tool to present fact-based information in a transparent manner that is designed to support an action to address a specific problem.

The CtD tool consists of three primary "dots": science, ethics, and history that surround a desired action. The dots may be augmented, depending on the topic or need to delve deeper into a specific area. The four areas are discussed in more detail below. The three dots (science, ethics, and history) were chosen because they represent general areas of content that are helpful, if not necessary, to consider with developing an approach to a problem. Legal considerations were not included because laws and regulations are often captured in a review of history and may be further addressed and explored once an action is identified. Another topic, or dot, that might be considered, may be economics, which is often an important consideration in developing approaches to problems. While economics is not specifically included in the proposed CtD framework, the model is meant to be flexible and the inclusion of additional dots is encouraged while maintaining a concise presentation of the most relevant issues. The information collected should address the identified problem, be supportive of a suggested action, and should be parsimoniously presented in no more than four written pages (two pages back to back) in order to recognize the limited time policymakers have to review information. If this compiled information is used in testimony in front of a government committee, it needs to brief but as complete as possible.

The connecting the dots (CtD) process

The CtD process is designed to apply a standardized approach to address an identified problem and support a specific action. The four pages of a CtD factsheet include a cover page with overview points followed by three pages that provide supporting details for action goal, including sections on the science, history (including relevant regulatory standards), and ethics. The CtD process really starts with acknowledging that there is a problem that needs to be addressed. Typically, this requires research into the scientific facts, history, and ethics. This generally leads to a first draft of action statement and the CtD factsheets. The first page is meant to provide a very brief summary of the stated problem and an introduction to key points. In developing and using CtD factsheets, users can specifically educate decision-makers, policymakers, and the public, which may help lead to a consensus for action to address an environmental or human health challenge. The front-page bullet points are meant to provide highlights of the issue, identify a specific action goal, and provide a brief justification for the specified action. The remaining three pages provide information on the science, ethics, and history, including current regulatory standards if applicable, and references. It may be further tailored to meet the needs of particular audiences, such as regulators, public interest groups, members of the public, academics, legislators, or legislative staff (Legislature, 2019).

The process of developing and using the CtD process is also meant to stimulate critical thinking about a problem and proposed approach to addressing the issue. The process starts with clearly articulating the problem and proceeds to doing research on the science, history, and ethics which leads to formulation of the action. Developing an action is really an evolving and iterative process. Some of the questions that might arise by undertaking this process might include: What are the underlying scientific findings? What were some of the precipitating events that lead to the problem? Who are the vulnerable populations? Who is or has benefited from the current status? Why should that be changed? Thus, how the information, past positions, values of stakeholders, and vested interests interact and connect is integral to decision-making.

It is also important to consider the type of target audience, or the intended recipients, of the CtD factsheet. Once the general structure of science, history, and ethics are addressed the CtD factsheet can be modified to suite a specific audience or presentation. For example, a CtD factsheet directed toward the general public may have slightly different language than a CtD factsheet directed toward legislative policymakers. For example, the ethics or history dot may be expanded to include more information on policy approaches over the past few decades. The CtD process is meant to be flexible and easily adaptable to different situations or audiences.

The author of a CtD factsheet has several important responsibilities. One of the most important considerations is to know the audience. For example, the knowledge base of students is very different from a group of scientists. One should also consider and acknowledge the personal biases and conflicts of interest or relevant financial relationships of the authors (Maurissen et al., 2005).

Three example CtD factsheets are included in the appendix (childhood lead exposure, lead shooting ranges, and fluoride). CtD factsheets also are being developed for many of the chapters of the book "A Small Dose of Toxicology" and will be available on the website www.asmalldoseoftoxicology.org.

First, a word about risk assessment and risk communication

Risk assessment and risk management has been around for 1,000s of years; after all, it was important to judge the probability of becoming a meal of the resident saber tooth tiger (Aven, 2016). The last 100 years have seen risk assessment and risk management become a recognized science (Hansson & Aven, 2014). The U.S. Environmental Protection Agency (EPA) has been using risk assessment modeling since the mid-1970s as a process to estimate the human health risk of cancer from exposure to pesticides and other chemicals (Embry et al., 2014; Faustman & Omenn, 2013). Risk assessment methods and related risk communication strategies are increasingly being pushed to evaluate and discuss very low-level effects (Gwinn et al., 2017). Risk assessment has been touted as the gold standard for setting regulatory limits to protect human health and is widely used in the United States and elsewhere. The process involves four basic steps: (1) hazard identification, (2) dose–response assessment, (3) exposure assessment, and (4) risk characterization (Faustman & Omenn, 2013).

> **Hazard Identification** Examines whether a stressor has the potential to cause harm to humans and/or ecological systems, and if so, under what circumstances. **Dose-Response Assessment** considers the numerical relationship between exposure and effects. **Exposure Assessment** looks at data related to frequency, duration, and concentration of exposure. And, **Risk Characterization** examines how well data support conclusions about the nature of the health risk from exposure. This process involves making assumptions about the probability of various conditions or characteristics being present with little or no relationship to the actual people or communities who are trying to use the guidance.
>
> (NRC, 1983)

While this approach is laudable and better than not considering these basic conditions at all, it is incomplete and outdated. What are not considered in this process are health outcomes other than cancer, such as reproductive, neurotoxic, developmental, and immunologic disorders. Nor are individual susceptibilities, preexisting conditions, gender, or genetic predisposition considered in this process. The unique susceptibilities of the very young or fragile elderly are not considered. The interactive effects of exposure to several compounds or environmental stressors are not considered. Nor are the health effects of chemical mixtures considered. Unfortunately, the U.S. EPA risk assessment process often is a permission to pollute with the implication that exposures at the level assigned by risk assessment are 'safe' regardless of the unique exposures or underlying health issues of the individual or communities exposed. And equally important is the fact that the assumptions and incomplete data upon which a risk assessment is based are poorly or not communicated at all to the public. As William Ruckelshaus (the first administrator of the EAP) once said, "We should remember that risk assessment data can be like the captured spy: If you torture it long enough, it will tell you anything you want to know." A new approach is needed. Risk assessment asks, "How much harm can we tolerate?," instead of focusing on the actions we should take to reduce human and ecological harm (Gilbert, 2005).

Beyond risk assessment

Current biological and toxicological knowledge now allows us to look beyond basic risk assessment in our effort to protect human and environmental health. It is time to consider whether or not risk assessment, as it is currently applied, meets the needs of the community and the new demands of chemical regulation. One demand that must be met concerns Environmental Justice (EJ) defined by the EPA as the "fair treatment and meaningful involvement of all people regardless of race, color, national origin, or income with respect to the development, implementation and enforcement of environmental laws, regulations and policies" (Eaton & Gilbert, 2013). Given the uncertainties surrounding the EPA risk assessment models and the possible adverse, noncancerous, consequences of exposures to harmful compounds, a more precautionary approach is needed. The foundation of CtD was built with a desire to strengthen the fundamentals of the toxicological sciences, risk assessment, ethics, and other essential elements of how we define harm (Eaton & Gilbert, 2013).

When chemical exposures yield noncancerous outcomes that are sometime subtle or differentially affect vulnerable populations, the precautionary principle should be incorporated in the review of the science. The most widely accepted definition of the precautionary principle is from the Wingspread Conference of 1998: "When an activity raises threats of harm to human health or the environment, precautionary measures should be taken even if some cause and effect relationships are not fully established scientifically" (Raffensperger & Tickner, 1999). Central components of the precautionary principle include the following: establishing public health goals; taking preventive action in the face of uncertainty; shifting the burden of responsibility (proof) to the proponents of an activity; exploring a wide range of alternatives to possibly harmful actions; and increasing public participation in decision-making (Gilbert, 2005).

Broadly defined, the goal of a precautionary assessment is to allow communities and individuals to incorporate the unique needs and challenges of specific communities and to include their values into a more comprehensive evaluation of a hazardous condition. It combines the philosophy and ethics of the precautionary principle with a standard scientific evaluation of the hazards. A precautionary assessment contains three basic elements: (a) community and social issues, (b) exposure, and (c) hazard and toxicity. Each element is broken down into a series of questions that are scored numerically and summed to produce a summary score for each element. In contrast to the traditional risk assessment, a precautionary approach is a more comprehensive and contextual way to evaluate the human and environmental health risks.

Recent scientific advances in our understanding of how DNA expression can be modified by environmental conditions, such as diet or stress, indicate that there are subtle changes in health outcomes. This is known as "epigenetics." In keeping with the acknowledgment of the interactive and combined effect of genetics and environment, we suggest that a precautionary approach to risk assessment is a tool to implement the ethics of "epiprecaution." A precautionary assessment moves beyond the usual risk assessment approach to include the ethical construct to not only reduce risk by "doing no harm" or "minimize harm" but also move to "doing good." We have an ethical responsibility to our children to have an environment that is supportive and nurturing and one in which they can reach and maintain their full potential, not just one that is free from exposure to chemicals (Gilbert, 2015).

Developing a 'connecting the dots' factsheet

Science—the bedrock of knowledge

Science is an ongoing and continual process that builds knowledge and facts following a systematic study of testable predictions. The scientific method is well described and agreed upon by the scientific community; it is the systematic observation and experimentation to test a prediction of hypothesis. The *Oxford Dictionaries Online* define the scientific method as "a method or procedure that has characterized natural science since the 17th century, consisting in systematic observation, measurement, and experiment, and the formulation, testing, and modification of hypotheses." Scientific findings are divided into many categories and subcategories as knowledge has expanded and continues to evolve. To this list can be added the life sciences such as biology and then toxicology. Disciplines such as medicine and toxicology are often considered to be applied sciences that use the scientific method. When there is controversy regarding the interpretation of scientific findings, it is important to develop an agreed-upon process for examining the scientific information or at the very least understand why there is disagreement.

Over the past few years the "sciences" have been used to justify a variety of personal opinions. Some have focused on the uncertainty inherent in science as a strategy to discount science or deflect the use of science in policy decisions. While it is true that the very nature of the scientific method includes the recognition of uncertainty, in fact, one of the beauties of science is that quest for knowledge is always evolving. Scientific findings, like most human endeavors, are influenced to some degree by the biases of the scientists conducting the research and the individuals interpreting published findings. More effort is needed to transparently acknowledge individual biases, conflicts of interest, and research funding sources. The toxicological science was not immune from labeling, and there developed a branch called evidence-based toxicology (Eaton & Gilbert, 2013; Faustman & Omenn, 2013; Silbergeld & Scherer, 2013; Stephens et al., 2013). The toxicological sciences are particularly susceptible to controversy about particular findings because of the money that can be made, or lost, from the way scientific findings are interpreted and used by profit-making companies (Maurissen et al., 2005).

Typically, any scientific discipline can be broken down to a common set of studies with defined methodology. It should be noted that toxicology is one of the few scientific disciplines that have developed a large and vibrant for-profit business that supports data development and report generation. Toxicology has both studies with defined methodology and studies with far more flexible methods that allow the exploration of mechanism of action and effective dose. These laboratories conduct a prescribed set of studies with primary variable being the dose of the test compound. The studies are done to determine at what dose an adverse effect is apparent. As a general rule, the greater the exposure to humans or distribution of a compound, the more well studied the compound and the larger number of ecological reports produced. The focus of the scientific dot is to summarize the scientific information that is accessible. Data or certain reports may not be accessible because they are not publically available and considered to be confidential information. There are a number of examples where scientific information has been hidden or distorted to facilitate conclusions about a product's safety to the advantage of the manufacturer of the product (EEA, 2002, 2013). It may also be a situation where one side of dispute focuses on uncertainty in the scientific process instead of taking a more precautionary approach as documented in late lessons from early warnings (EEA, 2002, 2013). These two EEA reports examine in detail the human life consequences of failing to take a precautionary approach in chemical management.

The last 10 to 15 years have seen many scientists working to summarize the scientific literature related to childhood exposure to an array of chemical compounds. These review papers can serve as examples of supporting literature for a CtD process. A particularly good example is the consensus statement on the neurotoxic effects of chemical exposure in childhood (Bennett et al., 2016). In addition, there are several authors who have a long track record of publications on the health effects of chemicals, for example, Lanphear (2015) and Axelrad et al. (2007).

Using the science dot

The science dot focuses on scientific data and reported findings of research related to the identified problem and possible policy or action efforts. For example, one scientific fact around childhood lead exposure is that children absorb more lead than adults and because they are smaller than adults, they receive a bigger dose for the same exposure (Gilbert & Weiss, 2006). This information can be used as part of the science dot and leads to an action to establish policy to reduce childhood lead exposures. Ironically the science dot can be the most difficult and complex to write because of the range of scientific research findings and the ongoing evolution of the science. It will typically take the most room and require the most referenced information. It is important to remember that you are building a story so that people can understand the scientific facts within the context of ethics and history and understand how this information addresses the stated problem and leads to possible action alternatives.

History—looking back to go forward

Understanding the historical perspective on an issue is a critical part of making good decisions. History helps us to understand how humans have shaped the environment and how the environment has shaped humans. But it also gives us a chance to learn from our mistakes and apply the knowledge and experiences that can inform current circumstances. The thoughts and arguments that went into current regulatory approaches to protecting human health and the environment are by nature historical, and, as time, culture, expectations, and science evolve, we can use these historical records to help make better decisions and take better actions.

Why study history?

History provides a framework on the basis of which we can better understand current issues, rules, regulations, and behaviors (Stearns, 1998). Understanding and using historical discoveries, reports, and experiences is an important, even necessary, element of implementing toxicological information in the present day. Historical references can help provide a foundation for current practices and policies, help predict future experiences, explain the evolution of scientific thought, and help us learn from mistakes of the past. Toxicological history goes back hundreds of years (Gallo, 2013; Gilbert, 2004; Gilbert & Hayes, 2006; Hayes & Gilbert, 2009). It helps us predict and even anticipate the future by reflecting on and learning from the ideas, and mistakes, of researchers, teachers, and advocates who have gone before. Understanding how things have changed, why they changed, and what stayed the same despite the efforts at change helps anticipate and even predict how future actions and activities will play out.

Often people from the past inspire us with their ideas, work, and thoughts about how they addressed challenges similar to our own. Reviewing historical activities for lessons learned, the ways humans have faced difficult situations, or things that worked well can inspire us to continue along similar paths and may even provide guidance in an increasingly complex world (EEA, 2002, 2013).

History is a study in trial and error and a view on what worked and what did not. Science too is a process of continual exploration and evolution of information and observations. Science and history both build on the work of the past to help understand the present day and even the future. Even research conducted 50 years ago can make important contributions to addressing current problems. Science incrementally approaches a better understanding of why things are the way they are and how things work. From this standpoint, history and science go hand-in-hand to help decision-makers continually progress toward better solutions to problems we face (Shaffer & Gilbert, 2017).

Relevance of historical toxicology

Humans have long been interested in how plants and minerals affected the human body, long before there was an actual scientific discipline called 'toxicology'. Human reactions to ingesting herbs, spices, fermented liquids, and various concoctions were often closely observed and reactions, positive and negative, were noted and passed on to ensuing generations. Experimentation and trial and error became the foundation for future advances as those historical experiences were passed on by oral tradition or eventually in writing. Even fatal effects informed future users; the father of Chinese medicine and pharmacology Shen Nung (2696 BCE; Gilbert & Hayes, 2006; Hayes & Gilbert, 2009) died sampling an herbal remedy—a great lesson for his followers.

One example of how history informs and impacts the present day is the use of the metal lead. The human health consequences of exposure to lead dust and fume were recognized more than 2,000 years ago with observers noting that "lead makes the mind give way" (Gilbert & Weiss, 2006). Despite this 'scientific' observation, future users of lead in metal-working, roofing, cooking, paint, gasoline, and ammunition often ignored this historical knowledge regarding the adverse health effects of exposure to lead, to the detriment of the lives of many. However, this evolution of scientific knowledge eventually influenced the regulation of the use of lead in a variety of products, though regulatory and policy decisions were often based more on economics and practicalities than health effects. It wasn't until the 1920s that lead-based paint was banned in Europe and not until 1978 in the United States. Lead exposure was found to be particularly worrisome for children as research increasingly demonstrated that lead exposure had a highly negative impact on early childhood intellectual development (Gilbert & Weiss, 2006). Unfortunately, leaded gasoline is still used in most parts of the world, as are many other lead-based products. Even historic uses of lead that are seemingly in a 'safe' form can have health impacts in the present day. The recent fire at the ancient Notre Dame Cathedral in Paris vaporized the lead-based roof of the structure, resulting in deposits of exceedingly high levels of lead fume and dust across the city and beyond.

One of the early practitioners of what is now called 'toxicology' is Paracelsus (1493–1541), a physician, alchemist, and astrologer. The classic (and historic) principle of toxicology, "the dose makes the poison," has been attributed to Paracelsus. This quote reflects the historic evolution of scientific observations that all substances have the potential to be poisonous, depending on the amount of exposure. In the 1700s, the understanding of the link between exposure and effect was advanced by Percivall Pott (1714–1788), who documented and reported that chimney sweepers, who were regularly and frequently cleaning the inside of Victorian England chimneys full of coal dust and soot, were susceptible to scrotal cancer due to their regular and cumulative exposure to the fireplace soot, or as the causative agent was later identified, polycyclic aromatic hydrocarbons (Hayes & Gilbert, 2009).

The scientific process and scientific understanding were not only integral to building a history of observations, discoveries, successes, and failures but have also put current problems within a context of years of evolution of scientific thought.

Using the history dot

Reading and understanding history gives us a chance to learn from past mistakes and apply the knowledge and experiences that can inform current circumstances (EEA, 2002, 2013). The thoughts and arguments that went into current regulatory approaches to protecting human health and the environment are by nature historical, and, as time, culture, expectations, and science evolve, we can use these historical records to help make better decisions and take better actions (Gross & Birnbaum, 2017).

History is an important part of making ethical decisions. History provides an opportunity to see how past decisions may have unfairly or disproportionately affected certain groups of people. The perspective of history provides a clearer view of who benefited, who was harmed, and what information did people receive when it came to making decisions. If people did not obtain sufficient, or correct, information or if information was withheld, then decisions may have been poorly made and the harm that was done needs to be addressed and changed with present-day decisions and actions. Without the perspective of history, many of these injustices cannot be recognized or modified (Lane et al., 2008).

It is important that we look back to go forward and consolidate our experiences into useful practices that allow use to learn from our mistakes. Using the opportunity to review the history of past actions, research, successes, and failures and incorporate those things into present-day thinking is a critical part of educating decision-makers and moving toward better practices and actions for everyone.

Ethics—a framework for decision-making

Ethics is a philosophical approach to considering concepts of right and wrong. As such ethics can provide a framework or guide to decision-making so that actions or policy approaches incorporate the values of the recipients, the proponents, and other concerned parties to an action. The ethics dot section provides an opportunity to explicitly explore the perspective, values, interests, environmental justice, and concerns (Gilbert, 2015) of impacted populations and individuals, identify who is at greatest risk, who benefits from the action, and at what costs (Figure 5.2).

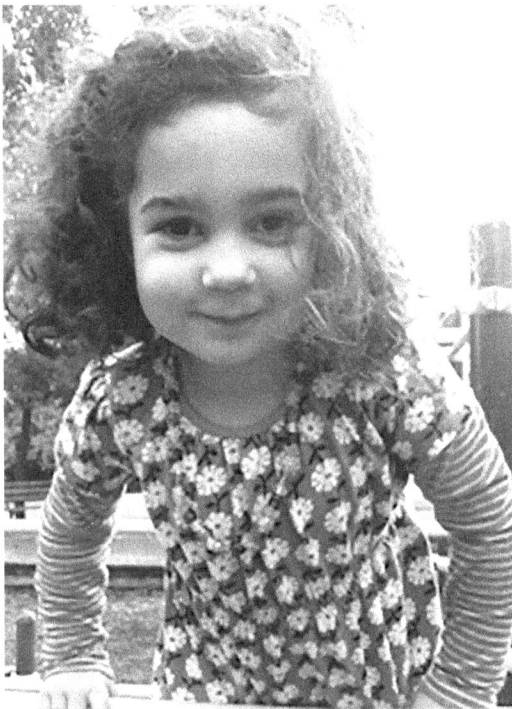

Figure 5.2 Six-year-old with developing brain worth protecting.

Why include ethics?

Consideration of ethics includes principles of conduct and how we choose to live. It identifies ideal activities or behaviors and includes discussions and consideration of justice and fairness. There are several approaches to ethics such as utilitarianism (a proper course of action is one that maximizes a positive effect), deontology (goodness determined by examining actions), consequentialism (rightness based on consequences), or pragmatism (moral correctness evolves); however, for the purposes of this chapter, ethics is considered to be a thought process that includes identification of values and how they related to the action goal. Governments use laws and regulations to motivate 'good' behavior; ethics implicitly addresses behavior that lies beyond governmental control. Some have refined the ethical approach to addressing environmental issues (Environmental Ethics; Brennan & Lo, 2016) or through combining ethics with legal and social issues into Ethical, Legal, and Social Implications (ELSI; Figure 5.3).

The fundamental ethical principles with regard to toxicology may be summarized as follows: (1) dignity and respect for the autonomy of human and animal subjects; (2) veracity, an adherence to transparency and presentation of all the facts; (3) justice, an equitable distributions of the costs, hazards, and gains; (4) integrity, meaning honesty and forthrightness; (5) responsibility, an acknowledgment of the accountability of all parties involved; and (6) sustainability, consideration that actions should be maintained over a long period of time (Gilbert & Eaton, 2009).

The more explicit use of ethical principles increasingly entered into policy discussions. Aldo Leopold, considered by many to be America's first bioethicist, summarized ethical responsibilities in a simple statement in 1949.

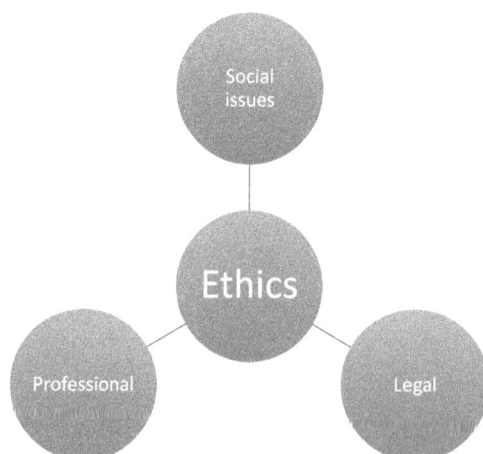

Figure 5.3 Dots around ethics.

A thing is right when it tends to preserve the integrity, stability, and beauty of the biotic community. It is wrong when it tends otherwise.

(Leopold, 1949)

Some believe that this ethical statement suggests that exposing people, particularly children, to harmful agents robs them of their "integrity, stability, and beauty," and indeed their potential, and is therefore wrong. Health, ecological, and ethical concerns about chemical exposures were highlighted by Rachel Carson in *Silent Spring* (1994), first published in 1962. Carson sounded one of the first alarms about the effects of environmental contaminants and catalyzed numerous regulatory changes related to chemical use.

It is the public that is being asked to assume the risks ... the public must decide whether it wishes to continue on the present road and it can only do so when in full possession of the facts …

Only within the moment of time represented by the present century has one species—man—acquired significant power to alter the nature of his world.

Rachel Carson (1994)

The idea for an Earth Charter (*Earth Charter*, 1997) was first proposed in 1987 as an approach to creating a broad ethical statement with the goal of establishing a global civil society. The *Earth Charter* took a step forward in 1992 at The Earth Summit in Rio de Janeiro, also known as the Rio Summit, which produced the 27 Principles of the Rio Declaration. Principle 15 defined the Precautionary Principle as an approach, and, some would say, an approach based in the ethical principle of 'do no harm' to protect human health and the environment. In January 1998, Wingspread Conference on the Precautionary Principle was held in Racine, Wisconsin to further define the Precautionary Principle (Gilbert, 2005; Kriebel et al., 2001). Many countries, states, and organization have since adopted the Earth Charter. Lessons can be learned from this approach when it comes to addressing problems and identifying actions related to human health.

When an activity raises threats of harm to the environment or human health, precautionary measures should be taken even if some cause and effect relationships are not fully established scientifically.

(Wingspread Statement on the Precautionary Principle, January 1998)

The concept of epigenetics also provides the scientific and biological foundation for the importance of "doing good." This concept could be called "epiprotection" or "epiprevention" to signify the need to move above and beyond preventing exposures to harmful material to one that is nurturing and supportive (Gilbert, 2015). We have an ethical responsibility to ensure that our children have an environment in which they can reach and maintain their full potential, which is not just free of exposure to chemicals but also an environment that is supportive and nurturing.

Using the ethics dot

A consideration of ethics and ethical principles when constructing the Ethics section of a CtD document encourages an evaluation of available information from the framework of values, identifying possible harms or costs, and obtaining input from all concerned parties with a goal of doing no harm to achieve the best possible outcome.

Incorporating an ethical component into the CtD document will require thoughtful development and articulation of fundamental ethical principles upon which the suggested action should be based. This approach may be time-consuming when working with stakeholders to articulate their values and goals, some of which may not be transparent even to them. It requires a move beyond what is legally required toward an exploration, discussion, and incorporation of the values of all parties.

Action—addressing the problem

A desired action is at the center around which to rotate the supporting information of science, history, and ethics, and other 'dots' such as economics. The 'action' dot works to address the stated problems and is the conclusion of the research and effort that went into understanding and linking the relevant science, history, and ethics. The Action is a desired effort to address or resolve the problem. A good example of this is the action of crafting a bill to be considered through the legislative process and hopefully will ultimately lead to a vote of approval. In this situation, the goal and audience are well defined. Another approach, perhaps a little more forthright, would be to conduct organized and structured research on the content of the three dots—science, history and ethics—to explore what might be possible actions to take to meet a specific goal or to determine whether a goal needs to be narrowed. The CtD approach is a tool for linking, organizing, evaluating, and communicating existing knowledge. The CtD can be used as a tool support advocacy for the action.

The desired action can be big or small but should be stated as simply and as specific as possible. For example, according to the Occupational Safety and Health Administration (OSHA), a worker's occupational lead exposure can reach 60 ug/dL before the worker is removed from the work place (Shaffer & Gilbert, 2017). A CtD action may be "Reduce worker lead exposure so that blood lead levels are less than 5 μg/Dl." Other CtD Actions may be stated in the form of protecting children from lead-based paint or passing a bill to reduce the use a pesticide. See the 'action' dot in the three examples in the appendix.

Conclusion

The connecting the dots (CtD) paradigm is designed to facilitate the systematic exploration of an identified problem and to communicate with and between the public and decision-makers. The CtD approach encourages people to think more deeply about the relationship between science, history, and ethics while supporting an action to address a specific problem. The CtD approach was developed with the understanding that there is tremendous amount of information available on a given topic but it is not often presented in a concise format and neither does it regularly capture the values of parties involved nor does it provide a clear rationale for a suggested action. By selecting highly specific examples from science, history, and ethics relevant to support the desired action, the author can keep the CtD document to four pages (two pages, front to back), which increase the likelihood that the information will be read and used by target audience. We need more time and effort placed in realm of scientific communication and education.

The CtD approach was developed with the acknowledgment that despite the complexity of the many issues, there is a real need to give people at all levels concise, methodical, and well-supported information to help them make effective policy decisions and take action to ensure a safe and healthy environment. The CtD approach puts scientific information in the context of history, society, culture, and values to help people connect the dots to collectively make better decisions.

Garrett Hardin in his paper "The Tragedy of the Commons" (Hardin, 1968) concluded that "It is our considered professional judgment that this dilemma has no technical solution." The vast majority of our problems in the complex world we have created must be managed or prevented. The CtD is meant to help us move forward to create a healthier world for all of our children.

References

Aven, T. (2016). Risk assessment and risk management: Review of recent advances on their foundation. *European Journal of Operational Research, 253*, 1–13.

Axelrad, D. A., Bellinger, D. C., Ryan, L. M., & Woodruff, T. J. (2007). Dose-response relationship of prenatal mercury exposure and IQ: An integrative analysis of epidemiologic data. *Environmental Health Perspectives, 115*(4), 609–615. doi:10.1289/ehp.9303

Bennett, D., Bellinger, D. C., Birnbaum, L. S., Bradman, A., Chen, A., Cory-Slechta, D. A., … National Medical, A. (2016). Project TENDR: Targeting environmental neuro-developmental risks the TENDR consensus statement. *Environmental Health Perspectives, 124*(7), A118–A122. doi:10.1289/EHP358

Carson, R. (1994). *Silent Spring*. Boston, MA: Houghton Mifflin.

Earth Charter. (1997). Retrieved from Rio de Janeiro http://earthcharterinaction.org/

Eaton, D. L., & Gilbert, S. G. (2013). Principles of toxicology. In C. D. Klaassen (Ed.), *Casarett & Doull's toxicology: The basic science of poisons* (8th ed., p. 25): New York: McGraw Hill Education.

EEA. (2002). *Late lessons from early warnings: The precautionary principle 1896–2000.* Retrieved from https://www.eea.europa.eu/publications/environmental_issue_report_2001_22

EEA. (2013). *Late lessons from early warnings II.* Retrieved from https://www.eea.europa.eu/publications/late-lessons-2/late-lessons-2-full-report/late-lessons-from-early-warnings/view

Embry, M. R., Bachman, A. N., Bell, D. R., Boobis, A. R., Cohen, S. M., Dellarco, M., … Doe, J. E. (2014). Risk assessment in the 21st century: Roadmap and matrix. *Critical Reviews in Toxicology, 44*(Suppl 3), 6–16. doi:10.3109/10408444.2014.931924

Faustman, E. M., & Omenn, G. S. (2013). Risk assessment. In C. D. Klaassen (Ed.), *Casarett & Doull's toxicology: The basic science of poisons* (8th ed., p. 25). New York: McGraw-Hill Education.

Gallo, M. A. (2013). History and scope of toxicology. In C. D. Klaassen (Ed.), *Casarett & Doull's toxicology:The basic science of poisons* (8th ed., pp. 3–10). New York: McGraw-Hill Company.

Gilbert, S. G. (2005). Public health and the precautionary principle. *Northwest Public Health,* 4. Retrieved from http://www.nwpublichealth.org/docs/nph/s2005/viewpoint_s2005.pdf

Gilbert, S. G. (2004). *A Small Dose of Toxicology. The Health Effects of Common Chemicals.* Boca Raton: CRC Press.

Gilbert, S. G. (2015). Ethical implications of epigenetics. In D. Hollar (Ed.), *Epigenetics, the environment, and children's health across lifespans* (pp. 327–334). Cham Heidelberg New York: Springer.

Gilbert, S. G., & Eaton, D. L. (2009). Ethical, legal, social, and professional issues in toxicology. In T. C. M. Bryan Ballantyne and T. Syversen (Eds.), *General and applied toxicology* (3rd ed., pp. 2815–2824). Oxford: Wiley.

Gilbert, S. G., & Hayes, A. (2006). Lessons learned: Milestones of toxicology. Retrieved from https://www.asmalldoseoftoxicology.org/milestones-posters

Gilbert, S. G., & Weiss, B. (2006). A rationale for lowering the blood lead action level from 10 to 2 microg/dL. *Neurotoxicology, 27*(5), 693–701. doi:10.1016/j.neuro.2006.06.008

Gross, L., & Birnbaum, L. S. (2017). Regulating toxic chemicals for public and environmental health. *PLoS Biol, 15*(12), e2004814. doi:10.1371/journal.pbio.2004814

Gwinn, M. R., Axelrad, D. A., Bahadori, T., Bussard, D., Cascio, W. E., Deener, K., … Burke, T. A. (2017). Chemical risk assessment: Traditional vs public health perspectives. *American Journal of Public Health, 107*(7), 1032–1039. doi:10.2105/AJPH.2017.303771

Hansson, S. O., & Aven, T. (2014). Is risk analysis scientific? *Risk Anal, 34*(7), 1173–1183. doi:10.1111/risa.12230

Hardin, G. (1968). The tragedy of the commons. The population problem has no technical solution; it requires a fundamental extension in morality. *Science, 162*(3859), 1243–1248. Retrieved from https://www.ncbi.nlm.nih.gov/pubmed/5699198

Hayes, A. N., & Gilbert, S. G. (2009). Historical milestones and discoveries that shaped the toxicology sciences. In A. Luch (Ed.), *Molecular, clinical and environmental toxicology. volume 1: Molecular toxicology* (pp. 1–35). Basel, Boston, and Berlin: Birkhäuser Verlag.

Kriebel, D., Tickner, J., Epstein, P., Lemons, J., Levins, R., Loechler, E. L., … Stoto, M. (2001). The precautionary principle in environmental science. *Environmental Health Perspectives, 109*(9), 871–876. doi:10.1289/ehp.01109871

Lane, S. D., Webster, N. J., Levandowski, B. A., Rubinstein, R. A., Keefe, R. H., Wojtowycz, M. A., ... Aubry, R. H. (2008). Environmental injustice: Childhood lead poisoning, teen pregnancy, and tobacco. *Journal of Adolescent Health, 42*(1), 43–49. doi:10.1016/j.jadohealth.2007.06.017

Lanphear, B. P. (2015). The impact of toxins on the developing brain. *Annual Review of Public Health, 36*, 211–230. doi:10.1146/annurev-publhealth-031912–114413

Legislature, W. S. (2019). Washington state legislature: How to testify in committee. Retrieved from http://leg.wa.gov/legislature/Pages/Testify.aspx

Leopold, A. (1949). *A Sand County Almanac.* Oxford: University Press.

Maurissen, J. P., Gilbert, S. G., Sander, M., Beauchamp, T. L., Johnson, S., Schwetz, B. A., ... Barrow, C. S. (2005). Workshop proceedings: Managing conflict of interest in science. A little consensus and a lot of controversy. *Toxicological Sciences, 87*(1), 11–14. Retrieved from http://www.ncbi.nlm.nih.gov/entrez/query.fcgi?cmd=Retrieve&db=PubMed&dopt=Citation&list_uids=15976187

NRC. (1983). *National research council risk assessment in the federal government: Managing process.* Retrieved from Washington DC.

Raffensperger, C., & Tickner, J. (1999). *Protecting public health and the environment: Implementing the precautionary principle.* Washington, DC: Island Press.

Shaffer, R. M., & Gilbert, S. G. (2017). Reducing occupational lead exposures: Strengthened standards for a healthy workforce. *Neurotoxicology.* doi:10.1016/j.neuro.2017.10.009

Silbergeld, E., & Scherer, R. W. (2013). Evidence-based toxicology: Strait is the gate, but the road is worth taking. *ALTEX, 30*(1), 67–73. doi:10.14573/altex.2013.1.067

Stearns, P. N. (1998). Why study history? *American Historical Association.* Retrieved from https://www.historians.org/about-aha-and-membership/aha-history-and-archives/historical-archives/why-study-history-(1998)

Stephens, M. L., Andersen, M., Becker, R. A., Betts, K., Boekelheide, K., Carney, E., ... Zurlo, J. (2013). Evidence-based toxicology for the 21st century: Opportunities and challenges. *ALTEX, 30*(1), 74–103. doi:10.14573/altex.2013.1.074

6 Developing teaching materials in ethics for chemistry and chemical engineering students

Tom Børsen

Introduction

International organizations, such as UNESCO's World Commission on the Ethics of Scientific Knowledge and Technology (COMEST), have for years argued for including ethics courses in chemistry and chemical engineering study programs. The arguments for including ethical elements into the chemistry curricula count that it could part of a strategy for securing sustainable development and betterment of the human condition (The World Commission on the Ethics of Scientific Knowledge and Technology, 2003) and that it helps chemistry gain a positive reputation, credibility, and a strong voice in the public debate (Benessia et al., 2016).

A limited amount of teaching material on the ethics of chemistry is available. Existing resources include Jeffrey Kovac's (2018b) textbook, *The Ethical Chemist: Professionalism and Ethics in Science*, and book chapters, examples, and cases in textbooks on research integrity (D'Angelo, 2018; Koepsell, 2016; Russell, Hogan, & Junker-Kenny, 2012), engineering ethics (Martin & Schinzinger, 1989; Van de Poel, 2011; Whitbeck, 2011), or environmental ethics (Resnik, 2012; Sandler, 2013; Vesilind & Gunn, 1998).

Systematic responses to the lack of teaching material in the ethics of chemistry include the European Chemical Society's (ECS) working party "Ethics in Chemistry" (Frank et al., 2011; Mehlich, Moser, Van Tiggelen, Campanella, & Hopf, 2017) and two special issues of *Science and Engineering Ethics* on "European Perspectives on Teaching Social Responsibility in Science and Engineering" (volume 19, issue 4) and "Ethics at Modern Universities of Technology" (volume 25, issue 6). Of these resources, only Kovacs' book and the ECS' working party focus directly on chemistry.

The lack of teaching material embedded in chemistry is a problem because successful ethics teaching in chemistry and chemical engineering requires contextual material for presenting, analyzing, and discussing ethical issues. Otherwise, the students might well perceive the teaching as remote and detached from their main discipline chemistry/chemical engineering—and reject ethics as irrelevant, not fitting with their cognitive setup, and meaningless (Zandvoort, Børsen, Deneke, & Bird, 2013). Without situated teaching

DOI: 10.4324/9780429318436-9

material, the future generations of chemists and chemical engineers might not be prepared for discussing ethical issues of chemistry.

This chapter addresses the lack of teaching material in the ethics of chemistry by reviewing a new collection of ethical case studies published in the journal *HYLE—International Journal for Philosophy of Chemistry*, aimed at use in university courses included in study programs of chemistry or chemical engineering.

Ethical issues in chemistry

The editor in chief of *HYLE*, Joachim Schummer, in 2015 took the initiative to issue a collection of "Ethical Case Studies of Chemistry" to meet the growing educational demand for material underpinning the teaching of ethics to chemistry and chemistry engineering students. He contacted the author of this chapter, who, for years, taught ethics to chemistry students at both University of Copenhagen and Aalborg University. Together, we edited the special issue with ethical case studies of chemistry. Three parts of the special issue have been published in 2016, 2017, and 2018, respectively. A last part was under consideration when this chapter was authored, and followed in 2020. All papers in the various parts of the special issue are published open access and available at http://www.hyle.org/journal/issues/special/ethical-cases.html.

Schummer and I justify our endeavor in three editorial introductions to the different parts of the special issue. Chemists and chemical engineers need to learn ethics because chemistry can contribute to solving societal challenges and to reaching UN's Sustainable Development Goals. However,

> real life solutions are never as simple as those for crossword puzzles. They always involve various advantages and disadvantages, improvements and drawbacks, opportunities and risks, to be discussed and balanced against each other. Thereby chemists are inevitably involved in disputes about values.
>
> (Børsen & Schummer, 2016: 1)

On the other hand, chemistry is often accused of creating societal problems:

> Chemists and chemistry students, if they engage in dialogues with relatives, friends, or acquaintances about their field, are frequently confronted with strong opinions. Isn't it chemistry that has produced poison gases, caused devastating disasters such as in Bhopal, India, and has regularly polluted the environment, and all that? How could you get interested in such a field? And how can you work for that?
>
> (Børsen & Schummer, 2018: 1)

Chemists must be able to reflect ethically, and they need to develop such skills during their university studies. In the introduction to the first part of the special issue we identify the ethical skills that chemistry and chemical engineering students need to possess:

- learn from pertinent historical cases of chemistry that have been in the focus of public disputes on how to avoid mistakes;
- conduct ethically responsible research;
- develop their own balanced ethical position that they are able to defend with ethical arguments and communicate to colleagues and the public at large;
- avoid being misled by corporate or governmental interests towards unethical behavior;
- help improve the public image of chemistry that revealingly contains elements of social isolation, lack of circumspection, and unscrupulous behavior.

(Børsen & Schummer, 2016: 2)

A prerequisite for engagement in solving societal grand challenges is to recognize it as an interdisciplinary activity. It has two implications:

First, chemists cannot address these issues alone; they have to collaborate with other disciplines, including natural, engineering, and social sciences as well as the humanities. Such interdisciplinary work requires an understanding of the possibilities and limits of chemistry from the outside, compared to that of other disciplines, i.e. an epistemological understanding of the science of chemistry. Second, interdisciplinary teams can develop useful possible solutions only in agreement with the norms and values of society. That in turn requires an understanding of the moral possibilities and limits, i.e. an ethical understanding of chemistry.

(Børsen & Schummer, 2017: 1)

Hence, the special issue is issued to fill the gap of missing teaching material for use in ethics of chemistry courses, and it provides "a canonical set of case studies to be enriched by more papers in the future" (Børsen & Schummer, 2016: 5).

Today chemists and chemical engineers do not learn how to engage in ethical discussions.

Our series of "Ethical Case Studies of Chemistry" is meant to overcome the speechlessness of chemists in moral matters. The aim is two-fold. On the one hand, chemists should, based on the best available academic knowledge, know better about the historical cases that have shaped the public image of their field. To that end, our collection comprises a canonical set of cases that every chemists should be acquainted with in our view.

(Børsen & Schummer, 2018: 1)

This chapter presents and discusses the main arguments of all the papers included in the special issue's first three parts. The call for papers to the special issue required submitted ethical case studies to address at least one of following aspects:

- Intentional misuse or misconduct
- Unforeseen local consequences
- Global and long-term influences and challenges
- Challenges to human culture.

These four categories and an additional one added later, Codes and Regulations, structure this paper's review of the contributions to the special issue. Hence, this chapter first presents the arguments relating chemistry to intentional misconduct and misuse and then it relates chemistry to unforeseen local consequences and so on.

An important distinction for teaching ethics to students of chemistry and chemistry engineering stands between the internal and external ethics of chemistry. John Ziman put forward this distinction 20 years ago in a lecture held at the Royal Danish School of Pharmacy (Børsen Hansen, 2002a, 2002b; Ziman, 2001, 2002).

The internal ethics of chemistry refers to the norms that hold chemistry together as an academic practice and is expanded by the values the scientific community of chemistry expects new practitioners to internalize. It is the answer to the question: What are you doing when you do chemistry? The internal ethics of chemistry overlaps with good scientific practice and research integrity. Its antithesis is scientific misconduct. It also overlaps with normative philosophy of science as set forth by Karl Popper (1962; 1959), Robert Merton (1973), and others.

The external ethics of chemistry regards the interface between chemistry and society. Answers to the question "Why are you doing chemistry?" are founded on the external ethics of chemistry that regards how chemists and chemical engineers justify/legitimize their endeavors. A justification can be ethical or unethical. You legitimize ethically your doings by referring to ethical values—ideal standards that you can compare your doings up against.

In the final discussion, I relate the papers clustered in the five topics to the distinction between the internal and external ethics of chemistry and, particularly, to one important area of the external ethics—environmental health. Despite this angling, the ethics of chemistry is not a subfield of environmental ethics. It would be a mistake to think so, as it would miss the complexity and variety of ethical issues that chemistry is embedded in. I extract some general insights from the five categories of ethical issues in chemistry: What ethical values are dominant, who has ethical agency, and how is responsibility addressed?

Intentional misuse and misconduct

This topic contains three articles: one on misconduct and two on misuse of chemistry in weapons research and development. The two papers on misuse deal with respectively the invention, use, and production of napalm during the Second World War and the Vietnam war, and Fritz Habers' involvement in chemical warfare in the First World War.

Misconduct

A paper by Janet D. Stemwedel (2016) deals with misconduct in a research laboratory based on the Bengü Sezen case from 2006. The failure to reproduce an experiment can be a sign of misconduct. The lack of replicability can be attributed to the following issues: the lack of competence of the person trying to reproduce an experiment; unclear, ambiguous, or deficient instructions; or falsified or fabricated results. The central point is that it is absolutely forbidden to fabricate, falsify, or plagiarize in chemistry and in science in general. It is argued that mentors/supervisors have a responsibility to teach graduate students good scientific practice. Does a supervisor hold a part of the responsibility for misconduct done by a graduate student? At least, it is argued, they have a responsibility not to pressuring the graduate student into misconduct by not tolerating failure. Costs are often related to disclosing misconduct such as being labelled a troublemaker or as incompetent for not being able to reproduce an experiment. This does not excuse someone from reporting misconduct if the accusations are investigated thoroughly and are well-documented.

Napalm

In Stephen M. Contakes and Taylor Jashinsky's paper on napalm (2016) the authors discuss possible wrongdoing of respectively Louis Fieser, the inventor of napalm, and Dow Chemicals, the company that produced napalm.

The authors use the principles of Just War in their analyses of responsibility in military research and production. This moral framework consists of two principles: *discrimination*, which holds that noncombatants may not be intentionally targeted; *proportionality*, which requires a just objective of war endeavors. Military scientists and weapons' producers should consider whether the weapons they are developing or producing could be used in ways that violate these two principles.

During the Second World War (1940–1945) Louis Fieser got involved in developing incendiaries, and he finally invented napalm. Contakes and Jashinsky's analysis of Fieser's responsibility focuses on determining whether he was aware of napalm might be used against civilians (cf. the principle of discrimination): Did Fieser anticipate potential large-scale use of napalm against civilians? They conclude that "Fieser first failed to consider anticipatable Second World War anti-civilian uses of napalm and then later even promoted them" (Contakes & Jashinsky, 2016: 39).

During the Vietnam War (1960s and early 1970s) public protests arose against Dow Chemicals' production and supply of napalm to the U.S. Army. The responsibility of the manufacturer reflects a judgment on whether America fought a just war in Vietnam, an assessment of the harms and benefits of the military's napalm operations, and whether napalm was "actually being employed indiscriminately against civilians" (Contakes & Jashinsky, 2016: 32).

> [A]fter an initial misstep in which Dow seemingly deflected responsibility onto the government, it addressed the Jus Bellum criteria [Just War principles] directly. It took steps to assess whether it was indeed supplying napalm to parties who were misusing it to unjustly harm civilians.
>
> (Contakes & Jashinsky, 2016: 44)

Fritz Haber

Joachim Schummer has authored a contribution (2018) that discusses weapons research in chemistry exemplified by the most famous representative of the academic-military-industrial-governmental complex: Fritz Haber and his role in the German gas warfare program during the First World War (1914–1918).

Haber connected these spheres by enrolling as a captain in the army, activating his pre-established industrial relations, and accepting an appointment in the war department that controlled war-relevant chemicals at the same time he was managing an academic institution: Kaiser Wilhelm Institute for Physical Chemistry and Electrochemistry.

Underpinning Schummer's discussions is a criticism of the current ethical debate of weapons research in chemistry that has so far only focused on weapons deployment and not on weapons research. Schummer's ethical analysis shows that chemical weapons research is morally wrong in both a consequentialist and a deontological perspective.

This was not at all recognized by Fritz Haber, whose understanding of social responsibility of scientists was very different:

> First, he argued that he had never cared about the Hague Convention [an international agreement banning gas weapons.] Second, he was convinced that in times of war ethical standards are to be replaced by patriotism, such that warfare engagement becomes a moral duty for scientists. ... Third, he was fully aware that his weapons program initiated an arms race among the enemies.
>
> (Schummer, 2018: 13)

Hence, Schummer suggests that chemical communities should stop honoring 'the heroes' of chemical warfare, which they do by awarding them prizes and by naming research institutions after them. Many chemists appraise Fritz Haber for his work with the Haber process producing ammonia out of N_2 and H_2 via electrolysis of aqueous NaCl solutions. Ammonia is today used as a fertilizer. However, in 1918, ammonia was primarily used for explosives. The chlorine that appeared as a product of the Haber process was used in a gas weapon—first in Ypres and later on the East front.

Weapons research is still a major contributor in terms of research funding, and the institutions, spokespersons, and practitioners of chemistry seem not to have drawn any ethical lessons from the First World War. "They thereby miss the chance of engaging young chemists in historical and ethical issues of their discipline and the chance to draw valuable lessons" (Schummer, 2018: 25).

Unforeseen local consequences

Three papers regarding side effects of medical drugs, chemical waste, and chemical accidents are included in this category of ethical issues of chemistry.

Thalidomide

A paper addresses the unexpected side effects of thalidomide—a sleep-inducing substance launched in Germany in 1957—that under certain circumstances as an adverse effect gave rise to malformed babies and hence was removed as an over-the-counter drug in the early 1960s (Ruthenberg, 2016). The producing company, Grünenthal, aggressively advertised thalidomide as a harmless drug, though at the time no standard procedure for pharmacological trials existed, and "the clinical studies used were far too short such that any long-term effects had insufficient time to develop" (Ruthenberg, 2016: 59). Klavs Ruthenberg, the author of the paper, cites Joachim Schummer for stating that those who create and prepare substances—in this context the leaders of Grünenthal—carry the responsibility for their impact. However, the paper notes, embryotoxic effects were not seen before and were a result of the unpredictable chemical properties of the drug thalidomide. Grünenthal cannot be blamed for not predicting it. Grünenthal's main omission was "the continued lack of reports on side effects [and] misrepresentation of the facts to the scientific community, physicians, and the public" (Ruthenberg, 2016: 71). The lesson from the scandal is that "[t]he dream of an entirely harmless but fully effective remedy should never be dreamt again" (Ruthenberg, 2016: 71). It is finally noted that the thalidomide victims should not be reduced to their disabilities.

Chemical waste

A case in the special issue written by Ragnar Fjelland (2016) analyses a chemical landfill located under the 'Love Canal' settlement near Niagara Falls. Hooker Electrochemical Company dumped chemical waste from 1942 to

1952 in artificial swales that were then covered with soil. The area was sold for one dollar to the school board of Niagara Falls with a disclaimer exempting Hooker Company from liability. A school was built in 1955.

The paper shows how experts disagreed whether Love Canal was a safe place to live. In 1978, the health authorities issued a report that documented the chemical pollution but assumed that the pollution spread homogeneously from the waste site. They concluded on that basis that it was safe to live in the part of Love Canal distanced from the waste dump. On the other side, the Love Canal Homeowners Association (LCHA) and associated experts argued that chemical pollution followed the swales shown in photos from the 1930s and linked it to the areas' disease patterns (geographical location of miscarriages, birth defects, asthma, urinary infections, and psychiatric cases). The LCHA turned out to be right, and the settlement of Love Canal was abandoned.

Fjelland recommends that experts collaborate with local inhabitants because "local knowledge may be more useful than mathematical models" (Fjelland, 2016: 122), for example, by establishing "extended peer communities," and that they are transparent and reflexive about uncertainties and underpinning assumptions, for example, whether tests have been made for both false positives (wrongful identification of a harmful effect that does not exist) and false negatives (failing to identify a harmful effect).

The Bhopal accident

Ingrid Eckerman and Tom Børsen (2018) address ethical issues of accidents at chemical plants by analyzing the gas leakage in December 1984 at the Union Carbide factory in the Indian city of Bhopal. It was the largest industrial chemical accident where over 500,000 persons were exposed to gaseous methyl isocyanate (MIC)—a substance used in the synthesis of the insecticide Sevin (Carbaryl or 1-naphthyl methylcarbamate). Between 3,000 and 10,000 were killed, and 100,000 to 200,000 suffered permanent injuries. During the cleaning of pipes water got in contact with MIC, the production tank began to rumple, and high quantities of MIC were eventually released into to atmosphere.

The cause of the accident was, according to the authors, the design of the plant, where "a dangerous but cost-effective method of manufacturing of Sevin was chosen" (Eckerman & Børsen, 2018: 34). Different pathways were available. The safest one—that does not involve MIC that explodes when exposed to water—was not chosen. This more secure pathway was used until 1973 when it was replaced by a cheaper production pathway using MIC. The MIC was stored in two large tanks, and not in several smaller barrels as was the case at Union Carbide's other factory in Virginia. The safety system in Bhopal was under-dimensioned and relied on manual operations—another difference between the Bhopal and the Virginia plants where the safety system was computerized. Safety expenses had been cut down in Bhopal, and on the night of the accident most of safety system was not functioning.

In the period leading up to the accident, early warning signals, such as regular leakages, had been neglected by the owners Union Carbide Corporation (UCC) and its India subsidiary Union Carbide India (UCI). After the accident UCC and UCI first claimed that the safety system in Bhopal was identical to the one in Virginia, but later changed that. Neither did UCC inform about previous leaks.

Even though they denied it, there is no doubt that UCC and UCI have a part of the responsibility for the accident because they operated with double safety standards in Virginia and Bhopal and because they ignored early warning signals. An accident was not a totally unexpected event.

The international community has to some extent learned from the Bhopal accident and other disasters. Corporate social responsibility has been codified in the United Nations' Global Compact scheme, the European Parliament's "Bhopal Resolution" calls for European companies to maintain safety mechanisms abroad on a similar level as at home, and UN, EU, and OECD support safety initiatives worldwide.

Global and long-term influences and challenges

In this category, we find case studies that discuss ethics related to global ecological effects of chemistry on the environment. It includes two case studies of chemical pollutants (DDT and bis-phenyl A), two case studies of different aspects of green chemistry, and finally a case study on chemical carbon capture.

DDT

This category includes a paper by Tom Børsen and Søren Nors Nielsen (2017) that analyzes ethical problems related to the use of DDT. DDT was intensively used during and after the Second World War to fight insect-borne diseases like malaria and as an agricultural insecticide. The use of DDT was restricted from the end of the 1960s until 2001 when its use was fully banned in agriculture and heavily restricted in malaria control by the Stockholm Convention.

The ethical problems of intensive use of DDT fall into three clusters: environmental ethics, human health, and the distribution of risks, benefits, and costs. The paper concludes that to prevent overuse of DDT, it should not be used in agriculture and its use in preventing malaria must be regulated. Hence, the paper provides a justification of the Stockholm Convention. It also suggests to enhance the development of holistic agricultural farming and the promotion of developing alternatives to DDT in combatting vector-borne diseases. It is suggested to set up early-warning systems that can identify unintended effects on human health and the environment so that these can be identified before they get out of control.

The paper's ethical analysis of the use of DDT identifies an underpinning uncritical belief in full human control over nature and formulates it in terms of the myth of Hubris and Nemesis.

> In Greek mythology, hubris refers to dangerously over-confidence in ones' personal qualities leading to behavior that defies the norms protected by the ancient gods. Nemesis refers to the revenging gods' punishment of the perpetrator. ... The myth can be translated into a relevant lesson for the use of DDT: undesirable consequences for the environment and society—Nemesis—arise as a result of uncritical and intensive use of DDT—Hubris.
>
> (Børsen & Nielsen, 2017: 7)

Bisphenol-A

Bisphenol-A is a compound currently used as an additive in bottles and other products made of clear, strong, glassy plastic. It is linked to diabetes, thyroid disease, cancer, and obesity. The cause of endocrine disruption is contested, as experts disagree on this effect. Chemicals' health risks come not only from factory pollution and waste sites but also from chemicals in consumer products. A paper by Abigail Martin, Alastair Iles, and Christine Rosen (2016) illustrates the latter source of chemical risks and shows how it can be handled by different stakeholders: regulatory authorities, producers, and consumers.

Authorities perform risk assessment that falls in four parts: hazard identification (e.g., carcinogenic or endocrine disruption), response assessment (usually tested on animals—but to what extend do animals model humans?), exposure assessment (where the substances are found), and risk characterization (determine what exposure levels are acceptable). Based on risk assessments, authorities can pass on regulations limiting or banning the use of a chemical substance.

Producers can substitute unsafe chemicals with safe ones, though the alternatives also need to be risk-assessed. Consumers can avoid buying products if their chemical risk profiles are uncertain.

PVC

In the first paper on green chemistry (GC), Alastair Iles, Abigail Martin, and Christine Rosen (2017) provide an example of how industry can make the production of polyvinyl chloride (PVC) more environmentally friendly using the principles of green chemistry. PVC is a plastic material used in durable consumer goods such as toys, credit cards, and interior designs. The wide use of the material presents risks to both human health and the environment. The ethical challenges derive primarily from some of the chemicals used in the production of PVC (e.g., chlorine, mercury, and vinyl chlorine monomers), from additives that make the material softer and more flexible (e.g., phthalates), and from burning waste containing PVC (e.g., dioxins and acidic gases) that cause problems for human health and the environment.

A specific focus is on how the industry can overcome path dependency and introduce green products. The paper presents the 12 principles of GC and discusses what can motivate the PVC industry to get involved in a green transition. It presents the most important routes of PVC production and discusses green alternatives based on biomass.

> PVC illustrates why and how applications of the [GC] principles can be gnarly in practice. The complex PVC production chain means that a single solution is unlikely to succeed fully: multiple solutions may have to be imperfectly patched together. … The ethical responsibility for acting may, then, be diffused across many industry actors that diverge markedly in their philosophies and capabilities.
>
> (Iles et al., 2017: 55)

Interdisciplinarity

The second paper on GC is a sociological study (Maxim, 2017) of green chemists and how they relate to the original 12 normative principles put forward by Paul Anastas and John Warner (1998). GC commits chemists to consider as an intrinsic element the health and environment risks of chemical substances and to collaborate with toxicologists and ecologists making GC an interdisciplinary endeavor.

> [GC translates] into an ethical requirement to consider the health effects of chemicals, not as a marginal or nonexisting aspect of their work, but as the primary aspect integral to planning research.
>
> (Maxim, 2017: 62)

Green chemists should be 'benign by design' by developing and synthesizing alternatives to dangerous and polluting chemicals. Hence, GC proposes that chemists and chemical societies should change their practices in three ways: by integrating impact analyses in the research planning, by collaborating with toxicologists and ecologists, and by designing green and safe substances.

However, interviews with green chemists show that a majority do not feel a responsibility for the health and environmental effects of the substances they design, invent, or synthesize. They also reveal that the prototypical green chemist has an instrumental perception of toxicology as a tool to determine the toxicity of chemical substances. They see the toxicity of chemicals as an external problem only marginally related to chemistry. The interviewed chemists express a similar impression with regard to ecology and environmental hazards.

The study shows a disciplinary divide between (green) chemistry and toxicology/ecology. Green chemistry is not an interdisciplinary endeavor combing chemistry with toxicology and ecology. Recommended initiatives to establish interdisciplinarity include:

> [J]oint workshops and conferences, funding for joint calls for projects and research proposals, and building procedures for sharing data between the [three] disciplines, removing terminology barriers, and creating joint journals.
>
> (Maxim, 2017: 77)

Chemical climate engineering

Dane Scott's paper (2018) on chemical climate engineering discusses scientists and engineers' contributions to solving the climate crises by involvement in climate engineering projects to capture carbon dioxide in the atmosphere.

Scott notices that human-induced climate changes push us "from the current epoch of predictability [and stability] to one of volatility [and uncertainty]" (Scott, 2018: 57). The effects of human activity seems not to favor human civilization in the long run: Anthropogenic climate change will "lead to famine, military conflict, and political instability" (Scott, 2018: 58), because crop production will fall, create much higher numbers of refugees, and make the affected areas prone to flooding, cyclones, and so on.

Hence, it has become mainstream to include climate engineering as part of the solution to climate change and its resulting challenges to human civilization. Climate engineering covers a number of techniques: solar radiation management, where solar radiation is reflected back into the universe by, for example, injecting sulfate particles into the stratosphere; carbon dioxide removal by adding iron to the oceans to stimulate phytoplankton growth; capture of CO_2 chemically, for example, by reaction with grained rock containing calcium and magnesium; and storing the CO_2 in biomass.

Climate engineering is labelled a 'technical fix': "a problem-solving strategy that reframes intractable sociopolitical problems as engineering puzzles that emit technical solutions" (Scott, 2018: 61).

The paper puts a special focus on the so-called moral hazard argument that states that it is immoral to engage in geoengineering because it will undermine political efforts to mitigate CO_2 emissions. The argument rests on the assumptions that climate engineering equals a hazard insurance, and people begin to behave more riskily when they have such an insurance. In this way, climate engineering will result in the neglect of initiatives focusing on mitigation of greenhouse gasses and primarily focus on the technical fixes. It is risky only to focus on climate engineering as the solution to the challenge of climate change. It is also risky not to do it and rely on political solutions that so far have not been very successful.

The moral hazard argument is linked to the principle of justice and fairness and an unfair distribution of risks—if climate-engineering fails, the resulting burdens will primarily be carried by the most vulnerable shoulders.

Challenges to human culture

This category contains two ethical case studies. They discuss respectively chemical enhancement of humans' capabilities and hyped scientific claims such as the creation of artificial life.

Chemical enhancement

Klavs Birkholm (2016) identifies ethical issues related to psychotropic drugs that affect the mind, emotions, and behavior. Around 8% of the Danish population used in 2011 anti-depressive medicine, most of them Selective Serotonin Reuptake Inhibitors (SSRIs). They are ordered for the treatment of depression, anxiety, obsessive compulsive disorder (OCD), shyness, stress, and posttraumatic stress disorder (PTSD). The ethical issues regard personal risks because the drugs do something to the brain. The drugs generate effects, but no one knows exactly what they are doing to the brain. Side effects have been reported, like addiction, dizziness, sexual disorders, and suicidal thoughts among children. According to the author, big pharmaceutical companies underestimate and hence misinform about the side effects of SSRIs.

The most significant ethical implications of psychotropic drugs are their potential effects on human culture: The high use of these drugs challenge the distinction between being ill or healthy. Is shyness an illness? Is it not normal to mourn over the loss of a parent or a child? The use of psychotropic drugs also challenges the human desire for recognition, which again is related to feelings such as honor, shame, justice, ambition, self-esteem, and self-respect. When drugs substitute these feelings, they also level out an important driving force for human achievements. In the United States, antidepressants are marketed as medicines providing self-esteem. The third cultural implication of psychotropic drugs regards human enhancement. The drugs can improve our work abilities if we are always happy, which is a personal competency in high demand at the labor market.

Hype

The paper "Are You Playing God?" by Joachim Schummer (2016) reports that Craig Venter—like many chemists before him—was accused of playing God after he in 2010 in a press release announced that he had created the first artificial cell in the laboratory. Schummer concludes that

> Throughout the 20th century, scientists, and chemists in particular, have publicly announced that they soon would be able to create life in the

laboratory. While this turned out to be wishful thinking, it revealed three important aspects of their views. First, because their predictions all turned out to be crudely false, their exaggerated views of chemistry's potential undermined their scientific credibility. [Second,] they all sought public attention for themselves or their profession through their predictions. This is further supported by the fact that most of them, I assume intentionally, confused the modifications of organisms with the creation of life. Third, in a surprisingly naïve way they transgressed the border to science fiction as well as moral boundaries by lightheadedly relating the potential fabrication of simple life forms to the creation of humans.

(Schummer, 2016: 156)

The paper argues that when the claim "you are playing God" is made, it does not stand up for ethical scrutiny (the ethical objections against the work of Craig Venter and others do not differ from ethical arguments against modifying organisms) but clearly reflects the general public's fear of 'the mad scientist'.

Codes and regulations

In this category, the editors of the special issue of *HYLE* put two papers: one on the code of conduct formulated by the American Chemical Society and one on chemical legislation in the European Union—REACH.

Codes of conduct

Jeffrey Kovac (2018a) suggests and assumes that formulating and releasing codes of conduct, a community—here the chemical community is the American Chemical Society (ASC)—sets ethical standards for how community members are supposed to behave. Members of the ASC must comply with the commitments stated in its code of conduct first issued in 1967 and revised several times—latest in 2007. Even though consequences for violating the code of conduct are not mentioned, the idea is that codes of conducts will raise the ethical awareness among chemists, not least if it is supported by educational material and addressed in chemistry teaching at various levels, and ultimately influence the behavior of chemists in the ethical direction.

The ACS code of conduct emphasizes guidelines for interpersonal relationships, for example, the employer–employee relationship or the mentor–mentee (the graduate student) relationship. It is inward-looking and concerned with the image of chemistry, though it recognizes the concern for environmental degradation. It does not discuss protection of whistleblowers.

The content of the ASC's code of conduct is compared to other existing codes such as those issued by the Royal Society of Chemistry (RSC) in the United Kingdom, the German Chemical Society, The Hague Ethical

Guidelines of the Organization for the Prohibition of Chemical Weapons (OPCW), and the Global Chemists' Code of Ethics convened by the ASC Office of International Activities.

All codes are aspirational and presented as statements on ideal behavior.

> Two important differences between the two international codes and that of the German Chemical Society, on the one hand, and those of the ASC and the RSC, on the other, are the emphasis on preventing the misuse of chemicals and on protecting the environment. Both the ASC and the RSC codes are silent on the issue of preventing the misuse of chemicals. Both contain statements on the environment but they are much less prominent.
>
> (Kovac, 2018a: 89)

REACH

Jean-Pierre Llored (2017) has authored a paper that investigates how the precautionary principle underpins chemical legislation in Europe—REACH—from 2006. The acronym is short for Registering, Evaluation, and Authorization of CHemical substances. The legislative corpus is a reaction to the fact that chemical substances have unintended and often harmful effects. REACH "requires chemical companies that produce at or above the level of one metric ton per year to conduct a risk assessment" (Llored, 2017: 84). If the substance is produced in a quantum of more than 10 tons it demands a full chemical safety assessment (European CHemicals Agency, 2016).

There are three types of environmental policies: A curative policy is undertaken when the environment cannot itself regenerate and actions are undertaken to repair it. When damage is reversible a preventive policy is needed, so that it can be avoided. Finally, we have an anticipatory environmental policy that deals with potential hazards. This type of policy is not about preventing damage from occurring but to anticipate risks posed by a chemical substance. REACH is an example of anticipatory environmental policy that is based on the precautionary principle. Prior to REACH, the potential impacts of most chemicals on human health and the environment had not been fully assessed.

Llored identifies three points for improvement of REACH: (1) REACH calls for development of safer alternatives to hazardous substances. This is more difficult than previously anticipated. Similar chemical properties often present similar hazards (cf. green chemistry). (2) Companies that potentially have vested interests in marketing their products are required to provide risk data, and this might conflict with the intentions of transparent and independent risk assessments. (3) Public involvement and the ability "to comment on risk assessment and socio-economic analyses are not precisely articulated within the decision-making process" (Llored, 2017: 98).

Discussion

The paper on misconduct addresses the internal ethics of chemistry and only peripherally deals with the societal effects of misconduct in terms of, for example, public trust in the institution of science. The papers on misuse deal with the external ethics of chemistry, though Contakes and Jashinsky (2016) argue that ethical reflections on anticipated effects of military technology should be embedded in military science's internal ethics.

None of the papers in the category of 'misconduct and misuse' have an explicit focus on environmental issues of misconduct or chemical warfare. They all deliberate on the responsibilities of individual chemists/chemical engineers, chemistry as a scientific institution, and the chemical industry. Hence, the present chapter addresses the ethical responsibility of both individuals and institutions. It also discusses the idea of a shared responsibility between individuals, for example, between a graduate student and their supervisor or between an employee and their employer.

The discussions on responsibility can easily be translated into an environmental health context: It is wrong to intentionally harm the environmental health. One only holds a responsibility if one has (or should have had) knowledge of potential or inflicted harm. One should not pressure anyone, for example, an employee or a graduate student, to wrongdoing, and everybody holds a responsibility to report wrongdoing even though one might get into trouble for doing so.

A case could have been included in the special issue that analyzed intentional pollution of the environment or intentional spreading of misinformation or fake news about chemical pollution. Some of the papers in the other categories cover this issue as a secondary topic.

The cases of misconduct and misuse all relate to trust as the most central ethical value at stake in the case studies presented.

> Trust is about the elimination of doubt in oneself, in other persons and in technologies. This ethical value commits a person or an institution to act in a reliable way so that others can trust in her or it, and treat her or it as an entity to be entrusted. A person or an institution must not say one thing and do something different.
>
> (Børsen, 2021: table 1)

Also, this discussion is related to environmental health. Science and chemistry should not be used to launch activities harmful to the environment by downplaying the harmful effects. That would definitely be misuse of chemistry. Another takeaway from this section is that chemistry should stop honoring chemists with questionable ethical achievements.

The no-harm principle is also a central ethical value addressed in especially the two case studies on misuse of chemistry in weapons research.

The no harm principle states that everybody has the right to be protected from harm, and safeguarded from illness, hunger, accident, and other dangers. This value encompasses protection from undesirable events and malicious actions. Sometimes a distinction between safety and security is made where safety refers to the right to be safeguarded from unintentional harm, and security refers to the right for protection against intentional harm (e.g. from terrorism).

(Børsen, 2021: table 1)

In this section the security aspect of 'no harm' is at stake.

Did chemists or the chemical industry know that their efforts contributed to harming civilians during the First and Second World Wars or the Vietnam War? This issue feeds into the discussions on responsibility that continue in the section of unforeseen local consequences of chemistry.

All three topics in that category regard health and safety effects of chemical production, which is a central area of the external ethics of chemistry. To manage external ethical issues new obligations are suggested for inclusion in the internal ethics of chemistry.

In "unforeseen local consequences," two out of three papers relate to environmental health though both contributions address it anthropocentrically as they are concerned with effects of dangerous chemicals (chemical waste and chemicals used in the production of an insecticide) on humans rather than on the environment. Hence, again in this section the ethical value of 'no harm' (and more precisely of safety, as the harmful consequences are unintentional) is central to all papers.

Here the discussion of responsibility continues but shifts its focus to the responsibility of unforeseen harmful events. How and to whom can we delegate responsibility for the unexpected? Different answers emerge: The thalidomide case argues that responsibility for the undesirable effects of the drug cannot be placed on the manufacturer, as they were not foreseeable. At that time, in the late 1950s and early 1960s, tests were not conducted to identify long-term effects of chemical drugs. The Bhopal paper states that the accident could have been foreseen and prevented if safety mechanisms of Western standards had been in place and in function and early warning signals had not been neglected. Hence, it is argued, the company held a responsibility for the accident. Both papers establish responsibility for not neglecting the existence of unforeseen consequences and for trying to obtain knowledge about them.

Humility is a second ethical value appearing in this section.

This ethical value is the anti-thesis to committing Hubris. One commits Hubris when one loses contact with reality and over-estimates of one's own competencies, does not listen to criticism and thinks one-dimensionally without giving alternatives any consideration. According to the Greek myth one will be punished by Nemesis if one commits Hubris. One is humble when one is self-restrained.

(Børsen, 2021: table 1)

In this section, we see examples of companies and experts committing hubris. The pharmaceutical industry in the late 1950s and early 1960s did not doubt the myth of a truly harmless chemical drug. Experts did not self-reflect on their models and neglected local citizens' points of view. To prevent harmful effects of chemicals from affecting humans this section suggests to strengthen and endorse safety legislation, avoid double standards, listen to early warning signals, be transparent about what risks the performed tests cannot identify, and involve citizens and incorporate their situated knowledge in risk management. The last suggestion reflects the ethical value of inclusion: "This value requires i/ simultaneous attention to the interests of all legitimate stakeholders, and ii/ a balance between this multiplicity of interests (including self-interests)" (Børsen, 2021: table 1).

All case studies regarding chemicals' global and long-term influences and challenges regard the external ethics of chemistry and are directly addressing environmental health. Three case studies discuss the long-term harmful effects of DDT, Bisphenol-A, and PVC. Here the no-harm principle is relevant. The focus is, however, not only on the harm inflicted on humans but also the harm inflicted on nature and ecosystems. The perspective is not only anthropocentric. Also here, the ethical value of humility is violated. The very intensive use of the mentioned chemicals is an act of Hubris. As a response to the problematic global use of chemicals, several papers in this category discuss whether and under which circumstances suitable alternatives can be developed and spread. It can both be the development of holistic agricultural methods that do not rely on adding chemicals, as in the DDT case, and the design of new and safer chemicals that can replace existing and harmful substances.

The section brings attention to how companies and the chemical research community can be motivated to get involved in a green transition as part of their work by developing new green products. The section discusses one seemingly appropriate solution to climate change—chemical climate capture—and relates it to the so-called moral hazard argument: that the promise of new green and safe technical solutions will prevent humans from acting environmentally responsibly because they give the impression that the problems will eventually be solved technically. So why change behavior?

Are new chemical solutions safe or green? It is here that the ethical value of precaution is brought into discussion.

> [This value] states that an action should not be undertaken if there are reasonable grounds for concern, though no scientific evidence, for it having dangerous effects on the environment, humans, animals or plant health.
>
> (Børsen, 2021: table 1)

The paper on Bisphenol-A discusses how authorities today perform risk assessment in the United States.

Chemists are not prepared for doing risk assessments or green chemical design. Or put in another way, the internal ethics of chemistry does not address such sensitivities. Chemists are not oriented toward ecology and toxicology, which are two areas necessary to relate to when doing green and safe chemical design or risk assessments. In addition to the proposals of the previous topic (e.g., strengthen legislation, establish early warning mechanism), papers in the section on global and long-term influences and challenges of chemistry suggest to develop new green chemical design and to work in an interdisciplinary way with ecologists and toxicologists.

Neither of the cases classified under the headline "challenges of chemistry to human culture" are directly dealing with the environment though both topics are, in my opinion, relevant for studies of environmental health.

The case analysis of psychotropics argues that widespread intake of such substances challenges human authenticity as they change our personality and turn us into someone else.

> Authenticity can be defined as the right to pursue one's own authentic perception of oneself. This includes the right to follow one's personality, rather than blindly reproducing the norms of society. Authenticity is an ethical value because every person has a right to unfold herself by pursuing what she finds valuable.
>
> (Børsen, 2021: table 1)

Similarly, one can argue that humanity's massive manipulation with nature removes nature from its authentic state.

The analysis of Craig Venter's work concludes that he grossly oversold and exaggerated his achievements, possibly to raise funding for his work, and that he in this way endangered public trust in chemistry. He referred to a culturally rooted fear of the 'mad scientist' to arouse public attention and promote his self-interests.

Similar mechanisms might be in function when tech-companies and other technophiles inflate and oversell technical solutions, or when the technophobe part of the green movement wrongly draws on public fear of chemistry or biotechnology to promote their agenda.

The two articles on "codes of conduct and regulations" complement many of the previous case analyses by reflecting on how to direct research and use of chemistry in ethical directions. Codes of conduct are a central instrument to maintain and transform the internal ethics of chemistry. Legislation is a tool often used to address external issues of chemistry, such as pollution and safety. It is important to include an active intention to protect the environment in professional codes of conduct for chemists and chemical engineers, and not only focus on interpersonal relationships, misuse, and misconduct, as often is the case. This is the responsibility of chemical societies and other institutions of chemistry. The final paper presents the European Union's chemical legislation. It explains how it works and identifies points for improvements. Legislation can be seen as ethics materializing on the macro level (national and international) and hence an important aspect of the ethics of chemistry. It links REACH to the ethical principles of precaution, safety, and security.

Conclusion

It is important to teach ethics to chemistry and chemical engineering students because it will both enable individual chemists/chemical engineers and chemistry as an institution to play a significant and productive role in solving grand societal challenges.

This review of the collection of ethical case studies of chemistry published in the first three parts of a special issue of *HYLE* concludes that ethics of chemistry covers different fields: misconduct and misuse, unforeseen local consequences, global and long-term consequences and challenges, challenges to human culture, and codes and regulations. Teaching ethics to chemistry and chemical engineering students should address all these topics. Global and long-term consequences of chemistry and their related challenges is the most pressing topic in the ethics of chemistry, as one-third of the case studies address issues in this category. A strong focus on this topic in teaching ethics in chemistry and chemical engineering is justified. This chapter also argues that the internal and external ethics of chemistry are entangled and interrelated. An ethics course for students of chemistry and chemical engineering cannot exclude one or the other of those perspectives.

The special issue constitutes the canon of the ethics of chemistry and potentially covers a full curriculum for a course in the ethics of chemistry. If the reader believes that a certain case is missing in the collection, they are encouraged to submit a paper to *HYLE* that presents the neglected case analysis.

The central issues in several case studies revolve around individual, shared, and institutional responsibility for wrongdoing and how unethical behavior of chemists might erode the trust in chemists, chemistry as a scientific institution, and the chemical industry. No harm, humility, justice, precaution, citizen involvement, and authenticity are additional central ethical values presented and discussed in the special issue's case studies.

It is suggested that the next generation of chemists and chemical engineers should

- develop new green chemical compounds and solutions,
- be critical toward hyped scientific claims,
- avoid applying double standards,
- listen to early warning signals,
- involve citizens and incorporate their situated knowledge in risk management,
- be transparent about assumptions underpinning risk assessment,
- work interdisciplinarily with ecologists and toxicologists,
- promote legislation on the national and international level, and
- promote codes of conduct among their students and peers.

Ethics teaching might indeed prepare the next generation of chemists and chemical engineers for the future.

Acknowledgment

Arguments promoted in this chapter have been presented on two occasions: at the 4th International Symposium on Ethics of Environmental Health at the University of South Bohemia, Ceske Budejovice, Czech Republic, held from September 9 to 12, 2018, and the 6th International Conference on Ethics Education at Spier Hotel, Stellenbosch, South Africa, held from October 3 to 5, 2018. The author wants to thank Friedo Zölzer, Joachim Schummer, and an anonymous reviewer for fruitful comments to a previous first draft of this chapter. The author wishes to acknowledge Joachim Schummer for his great work with *HYLE—International Journal for Philosophy of Chemistry*.

References

Anastas, P. T., & Warner, J. C. (1998). *Green chemistry: Theory and practice.* Oxford & New York: Oxford University Press.

Benessia, A., Funtowicz, S., Giampietro, M., Pereira, Â G., Ravetz, J. R., Saltelli, A., … van der Sluijs, Jeroen P. (2016). *Science on the verge.* Tempe, AZ and Washington, DC: Consortium for Science, Policy & Outcomes.

Birkholm, K. (2016). The ethical judgment: Chemical psychotropics. *HYLE— International Journal for Philosophy of Chemistry, 22*, 127–148.

Børsen, T. (2021). A quick and proper ethical technology assessment model. In L. Botin, & T. Børsen (Eds.), *Techno-anthropological contributions to technology assessment* (pp. 152–181). Aalborg: Aalborg University Press.

Børsen, T., & Nielsen, S. N. (2017). Applying an ethical judgment model to the case of DDT. *HYLE—International Journal for Philosophy of Chemistry, 23*, 5–27.

Børsen, T., & Schummer, J. (2016). Editorial introduction: Ethical case studies of chemistry. *HYLE—International Journal for Philosophy of Chemistry, 22*, 1–7.

Børsen, T., & Schummer, J. (2017). Editorial introduction: Ethical case studies of chemistry, part II. *HYLE—International Journal for Philosophy of Chemistry, 23*, 1–3.

Børsen, T., & Schummer, J. (2018). Editorial introduction: Ethical case studies of chemistry, part III. *HYLE—International Journal for Philosophy of Chemistry, 24*, 1–3.

Børsen Hansen, T. (2002a). Changing university science curriculum – To include philosophy of science and ethics. In T. Børsen Hansen (Ed.), *The role of philosophy of science and ethics in university science education* (pp. 91–123). Göteborg: NSU Press.

Børsen Hansen, T. (2002b). *The role of philosophy of science and ethics in university science education.* Göteborg: NSU Press.

Contakes, S. M., & Jashinsky, T. (2016). Ethical responsibilities in military-related work: The case of napalm. *HYLE—International Journal for Philosophy of Chemistry, 22*, 31–53.

D'Angelo, J. G. (2018). *Ethics in science: Ethical misconduct in scientific research.* Boca Raton FL: CRC Press.

Eckerman, I., & Børsen, T. (2018). Corporate and governmental responsibilities for preventing chemical disasters: Lessons from Bhopal. *HYLE—International Journal for Philosophy of Chemistry, 24*, 29–53.

European Chemicals Agency. (2016). *Guidance on registration: Version 3.0.* (ECHA-16-G-06-EN). Helsinki: ECHA. doi:10.2823/969. Retrieved from https://echa.europa.eu/documents/10162/23036412/registration_en.pdf/de54853d-e19e-4528-9b34-8680944372f2

Fjelland, R. (2016). When laypeople are right and experts are wrong: Lessons from love canal. *International Journal for Philosophy of Chemistry, 22*, 105–125.

Frank, H., Campanella, L., Dondi, F., Mehlich, J., Leitner, E., Rossi, G., … Bringmann, G. (2011). Ethics, chemistry, and education for sustainability. *Angewandte Chemie International Edition, 50*(37), 8482–8490.

Iles, A., Martin, A., & Meisner Rosen, C. (2017). Undoing chemical industry lock-ins: Polyvinyl chloride and green chemistry. *HYLE—International Journal for Philosophy of Chemistry, 23*, 29–60.

Koepsell, D. (2016). *Scientific integrity and research ethics: An approach from the ethos of science.* Heidelberg, New York, Dordrecht and London: Springer.

Kovac, J. (2018a). American chemical society codes of ethics: Past, present, and future. *HYLE—International Journal for Philosophy of Chemistry, 24*, 79–95.

Kovac, J. (2018b). *The ethical chemist: Professionalism and ethics in science.* Oxford & New York: Oxford University Press.

Llored, J. (2017). Ethics and chemical regulation: The case of REACH. *HYLE—International Journal for Philosophy of Chemistry, 23*, 81–104.

Martin, A., Iles, A., & Rosen, C. (2016). Applying utilitarianism and deontology in managing bisphenol-A risks in the United States. *HYLE—International Journal for Philosophy of Chemistry, 22*, 79–103.

Martin, M. W., & Schinzinger, R. (1989). *Ethics in engineering.* Boston, MA and New York: McGraw-Hill.

Maxim, L. (2017). Chemists' responsibility for the health impacts of chemicals: Green chemistry and its relation to toxicology. *HYLE—International Journal for Philosophy of Chemistry, 23*, 61–80.

Mehlich, J., Moser, F., Van Tiggelen, B., Campanella, L., & Hopf, H. (2017). The ethical and social dimensions of chemistry: Reflections, considerations, and clarifications. *Chemistry—A European Journal, 23*(6), 1210–1218.

Merton, R. K. (1973). The normative structure of science [1942]. In N. W. Storer (Ed.), *The sociology of science: Theoretical and empirical investigations* (pp. 267–278). Chicago, IL and London: University of Chicago Press.

Popper, K. R. (1962). *Conjectures and refutations.* New York: Basic Books.

Popper, K. R. (1959). *The logic of scientific discovery.* London: Routledge.

Resnik, D. B. (2012). *Environmental health ethics.* Cambridge & New York: Cambridge University Press.

Russell, C., Hogan, L., & Junker-Kenny, M. (2012). *Ethics for graduate researchers: A cross-disciplinary approach.* Oxford and Boston, MA: Newnes.

Ruthenberg, K. (2016). About the futile dream of an entirely riskless and fully effective remedy: Thalidomide. *HYLE—International Journal for Philosophy of Chemistry, 22*, 55–77.

Sandler, R. L. (2013). Environmental virtue ethics. In H. LaFollette, G. Brock, J. Deigh, J. Holroyd, D. Star & S. Stroud (eds.), *International Encyclopedia of Ethics* (pp. 1665–1674). Chichester, Oxford, & Malden MA: John Wiley & Sons.

Schummer, J. (2016). "Are you playing god?": Synthetic biology and the chemical ambition to create artificial life. *HYLE—International Journal for Philosophy of Chemistry, 22*, 149–172.

Schummer, J. (2018). Ethics of chemical weapons research: Poison gas in world war one. *HYLE—International Journal for Philosophy of Chemistry, 24*, 5–28.

Scott, D. (2018). Ethics of climate engineering: Chemical capture of carbon dioxide from air. *HYLE—International Journal for Philosophy of Chemistry, 24*, 55–77.

Stemwedel, J. D. (2016). The case of the finicky reactions: A case study of trust, accountability, and misconduct. *HYLE—International Journal for Philosophy of Chemistry, 22*, 9–29.

The World Commission on the Ethics of Scientific Knowledge and Technology. (2003). *The teaching of ethics* (COMEST). Paris: UNESCO.

Van de Poel, I. (2011). *Ethics, technology, and engineering: An introduction.* Chichester, Oxford and Malden, MA: John Wiley & Sons.

Vesilind, P. A., & Gunn, A. S. (1998). *Engineering, ethics, and the environment.* Cambridge and New York: Cambridge University Press.

Whitbeck, C. (2011). *Ethics in engineering practice and research.* Cambridge and New York: Cambridge University Press.

Zandvoort, H., Børsen, T., Deneke, M., & Bird, S. J. (2013). Editors' overview perspectives on teaching social responsibility to students in science and engineering. *Science and Engineering Ethics, 19*(4), 1413–1438.

Ziman, J. (2001). Getting scientists to think about what they are doing. *Science and Engineering Ethics, 7*(2), 165–176.

Ziman, J. (2002). Getting scientists to think about what they are doing. In T. Børsen Hansen (Ed.), *The role of philosophy of science and ethics in university science education* (pp. 23–44). Göteborg: NSU Press.

Part 3

Ethical challenges in radiation research

7   The ethics of the co-expertise process in the post-nuclear accident context

Jacques Lochard

Introduction

The nuclear accidents at Chernobyl and Fukushima showed that beyond the general concern about the potential effects of radiation on health and the environment, the irruption of radioactivity in people's daily lives and its persistence in the long term generate unprecedented societal and economic complexity. All dimensions of daily life are involved – health, environment, social life, production and distribution of food, amenities in the living spaces, as well as psychological, cultural, ethical and political dimensions. The result is a serious deterioration in the well-being of individuals and in the quality of the 'living together'. This situation raises countless problems for all social actors which call for difficult decisions.

In such a context, the actions of public authorities to protect people and maintain decent living conditions in affected areas are omnipresent. They mobilize, among other things, all the scientific and technical resources available, including of course those of radiological protection which are on the front line. As experience has shown, although essential to meet the challenges of all kinds that arise with the accident, science and technology are not sufficient to decide according to which principles it is advisable to choose between the different options which are available to decision-makers whether in the public realm or in the private sphere. It is at this level of the choice of what is preferable that ethical reflection is required to decide according to which values it is appropriate to choose.

The aim of the chapter is to describe the ethical dimensions of radiological protection decisions that become manifest in the management of the different phases of a nuclear accident. The first section outlines the ethical values which form the basis of the system of radiological protection recommended by the International Commission on Radiological Protection (ICRP). The second section presents the main characteristics of nuclear post-accident situations, emphasizing the human dimensions and their ethical issues. The third section describes the co-expertise process recommended by ICRP to respond to these issues as well as the ethical faculties required from experts and professionals who are involved in the implementation of the process.

DOI: 10.4324/9780429318436-11

The ethical foundation of the radiological protection system

The radiological protection system developed by ICRP was built during the 20th century by gradually integrating scientific knowledge concerning ionizing radiation, the ethical and societal values structuring modern societies, and the experience of professionals in the different exposure situations involving workers and the public. However, it was only very recently that the Commission presented for the first time in a synthetic manner the ethical values that underpin the radiological protection system (ICRP, 2018).

The primary aim of this system is to contribute to an appropriate level of protection of people and the environment against the detrimental effects of ionizing radiation exposure without unduly limiting the desirable human activities that may be associated with such exposure. This is to say that from the outset those in charge of radiological protection have to make value judgements about the relative importance of different kinds of risk and about the balancing of risks and benefits (ICRP, 2007). The difficulty is that there is no priority which is obvious in itself to make these value judgements combining science and ethics.

In practice, experience has shown that radiological protection decisions appeal to a wide range of ethical values which may apply differently depending on the context. These values all come from the three dominant theories of normative ethics which focus either on the duties and rules (deontological ethics) or on the consequences of decisions (teleological ethics) or even on the personality traits that lead the behaviour of agents (ethics of virtue).

As the French philosopher Paul Ricoeur has clearly shown, whether it relates to deontological, teleological or virtue ethics, the ethical objective is to ensure both the well-being of individuals and the quality of living together (Ricœur, 1991). It is indeed not possible to reduce ethics to moral questions, which he understands to comprise the rules which govern the process of living together. The ultimate aim of ethics, beyond living well with oneself and with others, is the desire for accomplishment. Ricoeur specifies that the desire to live well matches of course the moral obligations with their prohibitions and duties but that, in addition, the duties themselves must pass the test of wise and prudent decision-making in the face of specific concrete situations (Ricœur, 2017).

As regards living together, Ricœur emphasizes that it can only be experienced in times of distress such as wars or catastrophes. This is also the case, as we will see in section 'The co-expertise process', in the event of a nuclear accident which profoundly affects both relationships between the people and their relationship with the environment. It is indeed difficult to understand living together in times of peace because it tends to be blanked out, to be forgotten, even if it is a daily practice. It is only in times of tension and upheaval that the will to live together is manifested for and organized by those affected. Their desire to do so is reflected in the commitment to common

Table 7.1 The ethical values underpinning the radiological protection system (ICRP Publication 138, ICRP, 2020)

Core values
- **Beneficence/non-maleficence**: doing good and avoiding harm
- **Prudence**: in the face of uncertainty, avoid unwarranted risks
- **Justice**: fair sharing of benefits and risks
- **Dignity**: respect of individual autonomy

Procedural values
- **Accountability**: to be responsible for one's own action
- **Transparency**: to share available information
- **Inclusiveness**: stakeholder participation

projects for living together in a reality that has a long-term perspective, even if once normal conditions have returned this perspective will tend to veil itself again and fade away.

The ethical values on which the radiological protection system is based are presented in Table 7.1, distinguishing between core values and procedural values (ICRP, 2018). These values are intrinsically linked to the three fundamental principles which structure the system –justification of practices, optimization of protection and limitation of individual exposures. The following paragraphs give a brief overview of the values and their implications in the implementation of these principles.

The value of beneficence means promoting or doing good and that of non-maleficence means avoiding causation of harm. These two related ethical values have a long history in moral philosophy, dating back to the Hippocratic Oath, which demands that a physician do good and/or not harm. Beneficence and non-maleficence concern directly the well-being of individuals and at the collective level the quality of the living together. In radiological protection, these two values are combined together when deciding about the justification of a practice. The difficulty in implementing the beneficence/non-maleficence value lies in the plurality of options and the incommensurability of the factors and ethical values that must be taken into account to assess the damages and benefits associated with each of them and to decide about the best option. Attempts in the past to resort to economic computation using cost–benefit approaches have proven to be limited in deciding which is the preferable choice. The economic evaluation certainly makes it possible to compare the options according to a common monetary denominator but eliminates the ethical values inseparable from the decisions to be taken. For example, economic arguments alone seem to be insufficient to justify evacuating populations rather than asking them to shelter during the early phase of a nuclear accident. Such decisions also involve ethical values such as prudence, freedom, justice, which it is futile to monetarize.

Prudence is the ability to make reasonable choices without the full knowledge of the scope and consequences of actions. This ethical value has a long history in ethics. It is considered to be one of the main virtues rooted in the Western tradition developed by Plato and Aristotle, but it is also present in the teaching of Confucius, the Hindu and Buddhist philosophies, and the ancient traditions of the peoples of Eurasia, Oceania and America (Zölzer, 2016). Prudence is the virtue of deliberation and judgement, that is, the disposition to choose and act on what is in our power to do and not to do. In the radiological protection system, the value of prudence is closely associated with the principle of optimization of protection which requires that human exposures be kept as low as reasonably possible, taking into account societal, environmental and economic factors. This principle, which applies to all exposure situations involving radiation, is the cornerstone of the system of protection. It allows to take into account in all decisions aiming at protecting the people or the environment, the uncertainties of radiation science by acting judiciously and reasonably, particularly as far as low exposure is concerned (ICRP, 2006). In practical terms, prudence calls for vigilance and seeking to reduce uncertainties in the understanding of radiation risk. Concretely, this implies the requirement of radiation and health monitoring of exposed populations and the duty to relentlessly pursue research in the fields of epidemiology and radiobiology. It is the implementation of this duty that justifies the long-term health monitoring of people exposed after a nuclear accident as well as the associated epidemiological studies to provide information concerning the possible long-term radiological effects on the health for the exposed population.

The value of justice concerns fairness in the distribution of advantages and disadvantages among groups of people. It also includes fairness in the rules and procedures in the processes of decision-making (procedural justice). In radiological protection, the value of justice comes into play with the justification of practice and also in the decisions concerning the limitation of individual exposures. This limitation is implemented through a set of quantitative criteria (dose limits, dose constraints and reference levels) aiming to ensure that individuals are not exposed to radiological risks deemed to be not tolerable, taking into account the characteristics of the exposure situation in which they find themselves. In association with the optimization principle, these criteria allow also to limit inequities in the distribution of individual exposures in situations where some individuals could be subject to much greater exposures than the average. It is worth mentioning that individual exposure limits are widely used in regulations promulgated by public authorities in the form of standards and that they play an important role in the management of post-nuclear accident situations (see section 'The human dimensions of nuclear accidents').

The value of dignity is associated to the idea that something is due to a person because she or he is human. It means that every individual deserves unconditional respect, whatever their age, sex, health, social condition, ethnic origin and religion, and as such is considered as an attribute of the human condition. It is the cornerstone of the Charter of the UN (UN, 1945). The respect for human dignity was first introduced in radiological protection in the context of medical applications of radiation with the concepts of 'informed consent' in biomedical research (ICRP, 1992) and 'right to know' in relation to pregnancy and medical radiation. It was only with experience of managing sites contaminated by past military activities in the United States and the long-term consequences of the Chernobyl accident that the idea of involving those affected by radiation in their daily life has been integrated into the radiological protection system (IAEA, 2000). The involvement of stakeholders in a given exposure situation is now an integral part of the implementation of protection optimization. Furthermore, personal autonomy, as a corollary of human dignity, is now promoted by the ICRP through the empowerment of individuals so that they can make informed decisions related to their self-protection and also participate in collective decision-making concerning protection of society (ICRP, 2020; see Section 'The co-expertise process').

In summary, the core values underlying the radiological protection system help to inform choices in terms of protection, with the objective of doing more good than harm, of doing the best to reduce risks, of seeking a fair distribution of exposures, and also to treat people with respect. In addition, the procedural values of accountability, transparency and inclusiveness reflect the importance of assigning responsibilities to those involved in decision-making and the implementation of protective actions, in order not only to provide good information but also to preserve the autonomy and dignity of people potentially or actually exposed to radiation and also to protect the environment.

It should be noted that since ICRP published the ethical values which form the basis of the radiological protection system, it has been suggested that additional values might have been mentioned, such as sustainability for example, which can be already found in ICRP Publication 91 on the protection of the environment (ICRP, 2003). The most interesting suggestion is certainly that of adding the value of empathy, which is decisive for engaging those affected by radiation in the process of co-expertise as illustrated in section 'The co-expertise process' (Zölzer and Zölzer, 2020).

The human dimensions of nuclear accidents

The sudden irruption of radioactivity into everyone's familiar environment in the event of a nuclear accident is something that profoundly impacts the private sphere and raises many questions and concerns in the population, in particular among mothers of young children. Unknown to most, and in the absence of previous experience, the situation resulting from the accident is very difficult to grasp for non-specialists. The jargon of the experts is incomprehensible to ordinary people. In addition, the contradictory views of experts, reinforced by the media and social mobilization, contribute to the social amplification of the perception of risk, which may result in anxiety, stress or even fear in some people (Kasperson et al., 1988).

At the individual level, the psychological, emotional, symbolic, ethical and aesthetic dimensions of everyday life are affected, as well as, at the collective level, social life, production, distribution and consumption of food and commodities, the environment and so on. Not only all the local actors of the affected territories are concerned (residents, authorities, professionals, public and private organizations, companies etc.) but also a multitude of national actors who must face the repercussions of the accident and its consequences in their daily lives.

In addition, the presence of radioactivity strongly destabilizes relationships between people, as well as their relationship with their environment and their homeland. A difference immediately sets in between affected and unaffected areas, which not only discriminates against people who have been exposed but also against areas and products. The inhabitants of the affected areas feel this discrimination very strongly. Young people from the affected areas for example are perceived by the non-affected people from the rest of the country as unfit to marry in the future. The environment and in particular foodstuffs are perceived as dangerous, and goods and products manufactured in the affected areas are considered to be of lower value. Familiar environments such as gardens or recreation areas become hostile, and affected areas are socially and economically disqualified. The inhabitants of these areas have a different vision of the landscapes and symbolic sites than before the accident, and the common heritage is devalued.

The nuclear accident and its consequences also affect the collective memory of the nation. Everyone turns to the history of the country to try to give meaning to the event. Thus, after the Chernobyl accident, some residents of the contaminated areas spoke of the Gulag and the Second World War. In Fukushima, not only the battle of Aizu during the Boshin war was mentioned but obviously also the bombardments of Hiroshima and Nagasaki as well as the Lucky Dragon affair (Lochard et al., 2020).

The destabilization of daily life is reinforced by the many actions implemented by the authorities to protect people and maintain decent living and working conditions in the affected areas where the population has not been evacuated. Countermeasures to reduce exposure are intrusive and generate prohibitions. Radiological protection standards and criteria divide the world between what is good and what is bad and between what is dangerous and what is safe. Contamination measurements reduce the quality of things to numbers. Actions implemented by authorities disrupt daily life.

All these aspects generate a loss of self-confidence in those affected, which reinforces their concern over their future welfare and in particular the well-being of their children, including in terms of their children's health as well as in social and economic terms. The great complexity of the situation resulting from the accident combined with a strong loss of trust in the authorities and experts permeates a feeling of helplessness, abandonment and even exclusion among the affected population. Ultimately, the people concerned gradually feel a loss of control over daily lives with the feeling of being confronted with a danger without being able to assess the level of risk. Consequently, it is the dignity of each person exposed to radiation which is affected and which results in a loss of reference points and of autonomy in daily life.

The difficulties encountered by the authorities and experts in the management increase the feeling of loss of control over the situation. Authorities and experts are communicating with scientific and technical arguments to clarify the concerns expressed by the population and answer their questions. Thus, arguments laden with technical terms or unfamiliar jargon are generally not understood by the common people who then are forced to persist in their questioning until they are convinced that they have received authentic information concerning the risks of radiation. In such a situation, authorities and experts tend to put the blame on the population and adhere to the so-called *theory of radiophobia* (Girard, 1996). The affected population accuses public authorities of not only unpreparedness, delays, misunderstanding but also mismanagement, negligence or even abandonment. This also contributes to amplify social distrust and leads to very difficult situations as was the case in Soviet Union in the late 1980s (Lochard, 2013).

The Chernobyl and Fukushima accidents, for which the authorities, faced with the scale of the potential consequences of radioactive discharges into the environment, decided to evacuate the population from large areas and to implement a series of protective actions, resulted in a very strong disruption of daily life. They generated an unprecedented situation for humanity, giving rise to many questions and concerns among affected people: those living in contaminated areas, as well as those who have been forced to evacuate or have decided to voluntarily leave the affected areas. Each individual is permanently confronted with dilemmas: 'Should I stay or leave the affected area?' or (for those who left or have been evacuated/relocated) 'Should I return or not?' To answer these questions, people want to know, among others, the nature and level of risks; the means to protect themselves and their loved ones; and whether it will ever be possible for them in the future to live in decent and sustainable living conditions, including respectable lifestyles and livelihoods, as prevailed in pre-disaster times.

In summary, a major nuclear accident like that of Chernobyl or Fukushima results in a very complex situation generating many questions and concerns among the affected population (those living in contaminated areas and evacuees). In addition, the authorities and experts are discredited in the eyes of the population because they indirectly bear part of the responsibility for the events and they express different opinions as to the gravity of the situation. As a result, like the affected population, they are also deeply destabilized.

How can radiological experts and professionals who are at the frontline of the consequences of accidents take rational decisions and act combining scientific and technical expertise, ethical values and societal preferences in such a degraded context to restore decent living conditions for the affected people? How can they communicate effectively with all stakeholders and engage them into a fair risk management process respecting prudence and dignity? These are among the numerous challenges faced by those who implement radiological protection after a nuclear accident.

The co-expertise process

In its publication 146, ICRP recommends the implementation of what is called the 'co-expertise process' to communicate and empower the people affected by a nuclear accident situation in order to help them regain control of their daily lives (ICRP, 2020). The term 'co-expertise process' is an abbreviation for cooperation between experts and stakeholders. The notion of 'co-expertise process' emerged in the late 1990s in the context of the rehabilitation of living conditions in the territories affected by the Chernobyl accident (Heriard Dubreuil, 1999; Bataille et al., 2008). It has been enriched and refined in recent years through the experience gained in communities of Japan following the Fukushima accident (Ando, 2018; Takamura et al., 2018; Lochard et al., 2020; Yasutaka et al., 2020).

The Japanese experience also provided a better understanding of how the fundamental ethical and procedural values that underpin the radiological protection system relate to decision-making processes regarding radiation risk management in post-nuclear accident situations. It also highlighted the importance of the ethical positioning of experts and professionals in radiological protection to ensure the effectiveness of the recovery process after the accident (Schneider et al., 2019).

The co-expertise process was built gradually from an empirical trial-and-error learning approach during more than a decade. However, in the background, the process was influenced by the advances of the previous two decades in the development of risk assessment and management (UNNRC, 2009), particularly the optimization process recommended by ICRP (ICRP, 2006), and progress made in risk perception (Slovic, 2000) and risk communication (Covello, 2011). The process was also inspired by the reflections that came to the fore in the late 1990s on the governance of risks related to complex and controversial situations involving risk (Renn, 1999, 2008).

The co-expertise process attempts to meet two major objectives: first, to engage affected people in the recovery process after the accident, and, second, to empower them by developing a practical radiological protection culture so that they can make informed decisions about their protection and thus restore their dignity.

The process is based on four steps summarily described in the following paragraphs (see Figure 7.1). This distinction is to facilitate their descriptions

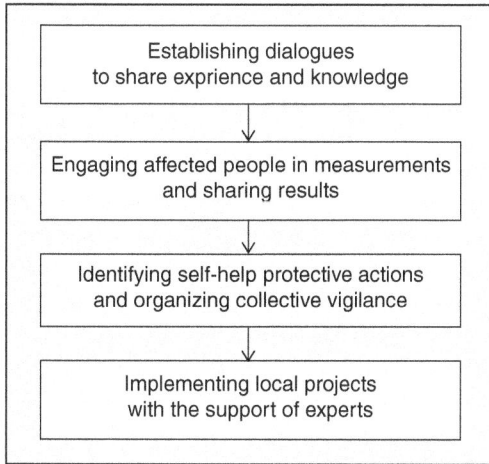

Figure 7.1 The co-expertise process (ICRP, 2020).

and roles. In practice, it should be noted that these steps interact with each other. If there is indeed a first step of dialogue to engage the local actors in the process and a second step centred on measurements of radioactivity in the environment close to people and the assessment of their individual radiation exposure, the following steps can gradually be deployed in parallel. Experience has shown that the process of co-expertise takes time, generally several years, as the people involved progress step-by-step in their understanding and their positioning in relation to the situation.

Establishing a dialogue

The first step of the process aims at establishing a dialogue between experts and stakeholders from affected communities to identify the problems and the challenges they are confronted with. To be effective, the dialogue must continue during all steps and beyond the dimension of protection, which is the major preoccupation of the participants during the first exchanges, and must gradually focus on the well-being and the quality of living together in the communities concerned. Through this dialogue, the affected people can have a fair opportunity to express their concerns and expectations on the situation at stake, share their experiences about their living conditions and ask questions about the situation.

Dialogue goes beyond the good intention of involving affected people in risk communication in order to inform them of the situation they are facing. The objective of the dialogue, which is based on two-way communication and takes place at the level of the affected communities, is to enable experts to understand the concerns of the affected people and their points of view on this situation and understand in particular the local specificities that govern radiation exposure through the elicitation of individual behaviours and habits as well as local customs and practices. The dialogue first allows each participant to understand that they are not alone in regard to their situation or their concerns, and the answers of the experts help the participant realize that their exposure depends on their living place, behaviour and individual activities.

Effective dialogue brings together various skills and sensibilities and helps to identify the real concerns and expectations of people. It abolishes the duality between the experts and the laymen, that is, those who know and those who do not know. It is a space to share experiences freely and openly and for everyone to listen to different points of view and opinions on the situation and to put themselves in the shoes of other participants. The use of common language and narrative facilitates the sharing of each person's intimate experience and the revelation of the richness of sense of the situation and also allows each one to revisit their values and aspirations and affirm their identity. The close relationships between the participants facilitate understanding the complexity of the situations they face and facilitate the search for solutions to the individual and collective problems identified together. To be effective, the dialogue must imperatively be based on careful listening and mutual respect of the participants. From this point of view, empathy is essential.

The dialogue allows affected people to gradually become aware of the factors and issues of the complexity with which they are confronted, but it is by intervening concretely in their neighbourhood, at the level of the community where they live, that it is possible to bring into play their capacity and their dispositions, which are essential to get them to take control of the situation. Regular exchanges between affected people within a community and experts not only bring together various points of view but also diverse skills and responsibilities that can be mobilized to deal with difficult situations. It opens up possibilities and avoids sterile and divisive face-to-face confrontation. It allows to get out of the scientific and political discourse which tends to confiscate the debates. The dialogue is for affected people who participate in it, the first step in restoring the dignity of each person.

Engaging people in measurements

The second step is to engage affected people in measurements of radioactivity, in order to help them understand when, where and how they are, or will be, exposed to radiation in their day-to-day lives. By involving affected people in the measurement of radioactivity it is possible to make visible what was invisible to them. Measurements allow the affected individual(s) to become aware of the reasons of their exposure and to look for possible protective actions to reduce or avoid doing things or visiting places that will expose them to radioactivity. To engage people in measurements should be progressively developed based on a comprehensive monitoring approach performed by the authorities and/or by affected people themselves (self-monitoring). By doing so, people regain progressively control over the radiological situation they are confronted with.

To be meaningful, measurements should be done step-by-step from sources of exposure to the exposures received by individuals through the various exposure pathways. When performing measurements, the most important aspect for the experts involved is to pay attention to the concerns expressed by the affected people. This allows to provide adapted measurement instruments to the stakeholders and to accompany them in the definition of the monitoring programme as well as in the interpretation of the results. The aim is for affected people to be able to think about the meaning and implications of the results of the measurements for their lives. The involvement of affected people in the analysis of the results of measurement and their sharing with others in their community allow them to identify the course of action to be taken for protecting themselves in their daily lives (Ando, 2016).

In addition, experience has shown that it is during measurements in which people interact with experts, that they become familiar with the mechanisms that govern the exposure of people to radiation as well as the basic concepts and units of radiological protection. It is also through this approach, which allows them to observe that the results of their measurements corroborate those which are otherwise disseminated by the authorities, that confidence in the latter is gradually being re-established.

Finally, sharing measurement results to discuss the situation of the community is a powerful means to allow each individual to understand their own situation and to identify opportunities to improve their protection.

Self-help protective actions

The third step in the process is the identification and implementation of protective actions by the affected people themselves. Indeed, by taking measurements together, the experts and the affected persons identify the main causes of exposure of individuals, that is, where, when and how people are exposed, taking into account the local situation, their daily activities and their personal behaviours and habits. With this information in hand, individuals are able to understand their own situation and identify opportunities to improve their protection. Measurements therefore allow everyone to make decisions to reduce their own exposure. They also make it possible to not only identify self-help protective actions implemented by the individuals concerned but also establish a radiological surveillance programme within the communities to favour the development of a 'citizen vigilance' on the radiological situation (Maître et al., 2021). Whether they are implemented individually or collectively, the support of the public and/or private sectors (experts and authorities) is essential to bring together the necessary technical and human resources.

Self-help protective actions are complementary to the collective protective actions decided and implemented by authorities for the affected areas after the nuclear accident, like food restrictions or decontamination which by their nature apply without taking into account the individual situations of the residents. The co-expertise process by favouring individual initiatives is a way to reinforce the effectiveness of the protective strategy of the authorities. It also allows to evaluate the effectiveness of the protective actions driven by the authorities with possibilities to adapt them if necessary. The experience gained from this process can also be helpful in understanding the meaning and usefulness of radiological protection criteria decreed by authorities to manage the situation.

The process of co-expertise is similar to the classic process of optimization of protection recommended by the ICRP. It uses a similar analytical approach to identify possible actions and then decide on the most appropriate ones. This approach is based on the quantitative elements resulting from the measurements and also calls for the balancing of many factors related to the feasibility of the actions taking into account the context as well and the impact on the well-being of affected people. Past experience has shown that once affected people engage in self-help protective actions, they come into conflict with their desire to enjoy life. Depending on the individual temperament, it is the concern for protection that wins or a reasonable risk-taking.

Implementing local projects

The fourth step is to accompany the development of local projects aiming at protecting people and also contributing to restore sustainable livelihoods in the communities. Past experience has shown that these projects in different fields (radiological protection, education, social activities, culture, memory, economy, etc.) should reflect the local situation in the communities and also contribute to improve the well-being of individuals and the quality of the living together of the affected communities. Progressively, people understand more and more the factors driving their exposure and how they can protect themselves. Consequently, they wish to take actions to improve the situation.

By developing local projects, people consider again the possibilities of shaping their future. This contrasts with the early phase of the accident where those affected did not understand the situation, did not know what to do and did not see a future for themselves. In this respect, local projects are important for those involved in finding a way for their personal achievement that was blocked after the nuclear accident. Local projects are the mechanisms to put people again in the dynamic of not only self-development but also collective development. It is the way to help people to stimulate personal fulfilment and also to create connection between people within the community and restore trust in experts and authorities.

About ethics

The co-expertise approach aims to integrate technical expertise and the values carried by the people concerned in compliance with regulatory requirements. The philosophy behind the process is that experts and stakeholders can jointly solve the challenges facing the community through their respective expertise – that of scientific and technical experts and that of daily human experience made up of traditions, culture and aspiration to live well with and for others. Local actors are a valuable resource not only for understanding the concerns of the community but also for deciding what actions to implement, because their interests are at stake. Experts are a valuable support to help gather technical data and assess rational options and their impacts. Affected people live with the consequences of decisions and are therefore the best judges to decide which options to adopt.

By empowering those involved, the co-expertise process develops a practical radiological protection culture which allows members of the community to interpret the results of radiation measurements, to build their own benchmarks in relation to the radioactivity present in their daily life, to make their own decisions to protect themselves and their loved ones and, finally, to assess the effectiveness of protective actions implemented by themselves or by authorities and organizations (ICRP, 2020).

Radiological protection is not an end in itself. The objective of post-nuclear accident recovery is, beyond protection, to ensure decent and sustainable living conditions in the affected communities. Rebuilding living together requires implementing local projects that help improve the well-being of individuals and the quality of social life. This is why experience has shown that the communities having participated in co-expertise experiments are keen to develop projects not only in the fields of radiological protection but also in education, memory and culture (Schneider & Lochard, 2021). To effectively implement these local projects, cooperation with the competent authorities, public and private organizations, and experts and professionals is essential.

Experience from Chernobyl and Fukushima has shown that, in order for experts to be credible, they must not only master the scientific basis of radiological protection and its practical implementation (Accountability) but must also share openly all information they own and recognize their limitations (Transparency) and deliberate and decide together with stakeholders (Inclusiveness). Here we find in action the procedural values highlighted by the radiological protection system.

Finally, the co-expertise process is based on the recognition that to make sense for people confronted with radiation, knowledge about radiological protection must be anchored to their daily reality to allow them to act to improve their future living conditions. This is only possible if they are directly involved in the post-disaster recovery process. This requires the mobilization of specific skills from the experts, what Paul Ricœur called the *practical*

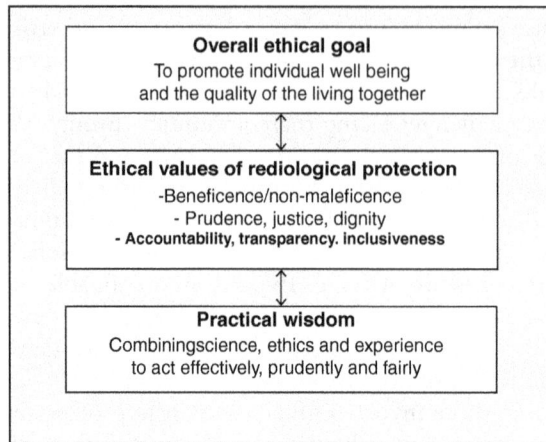

```
┌─────────────────────────────────────────────┐
│   ┌─────────────────────────────────────┐    │
│   │        Overall ethical goal         │    │
│   │    To promote individual well being │    │
│   │   and the quality of the living together │ │
│   └─────────────────────────────────────┘    │
│                    ↕                          │
│   ┌─────────────────────────────────────┐    │
│   │  Ethical values of rediological protection │ │
│   │     -Beneficence/non-maleficence    │    │
│   │        - Prudence, justice, dignity │    │
│   │  - Accountabllity, transparency. inclusiveness │ │
│   └─────────────────────────────────────┘    │
│                    ↕                          │
│   ┌─────────────────────────────────────┐    │
│   │           Practical wisdom          │    │
│   │   Combiningscience, ethics and experience │ │
│   │    to act effectively, prudently and fairly │ │
│   └─────────────────────────────────────┘    │
└─────────────────────────────────────────────┘
```

Figure 7.2 The three levels of ethics of the radiological protection system.

wisdom (see Figure 7.2), which makes it possible to put ethical values – here the values on which the radiological protection system is based – at the service of the overall ethical objective of promoting individual well-being and the quality of living together in order to satisfy the desire for accomplishment to which each and every human being aspires (Ricoeur, 1991).

Conclusion

The objective of the co-expertise process in the post-nuclear accident context is to seek together wise and prudent decisions aimed at promoting the personal well-being of all those involved in the process: the people affected, the experts, the professionals, and the authorities. One of the aspects of the nuclear post-accident complexity is that most of the choices to be made in terms of protection are not to be made between black or white, but between grey and grey, and even sometimes between black and black. This is true for collective choices (evacuation, food restrictions, environmental decontamination etc.) as well as for individual choices. People in the affected territories have to find their daily balance between protecting themselves and enjoying life.

The complexity generated by the accident amplifies the plurality of points of view and the antagonisms of the interests of the stakeholders which inevitably result in debates, even conflicts, among experts and authorities from which non-experts feel excluded. The search for compromise is the only way to aim for the common good when contradictory values clash. Compromise ensures that differences of points of view and conflicts of values do not lead to blockages in action, or in extreme cases, to resorting to violence in order to resolve issues. The refusal to listen to the arguments of others annihilates the search for the common good with a view to action.

The co-expertise process refers directly to ethical values, because it is in the name of values that it is necessary to act in one direction or another. The difficulty is that in a context of plurality of points of view there is no value which is a priori dominating. What is preferable can only be a matter of democratic debate between stakeholders. The idea that decisions about protective actions might be solely a matter of scientific rationality is an illusion. Of course, rationality is necessary, but it is simply insufficient in complex situations such as the post-nuclear accident context.

References

Ando R., 2016. Measuring, discussing, and living together: Lessons from 4 years in Suetsugi. London: SAGE Publications; *Annals of ICRP*, 45(1S), 75–83.

Ando R., 2018. Trust – what connects science to daily life. *Health Physics*, 115(5), 581–589.

Bataille C., Crouail P., Lochard J., 2008. Rehabilitation of living conditions in the post-Chernobyl context: Implementation of an inclusive radiation monitoring system in the Bragin District in Belarus. In: Proceedings of the International Conference on 'Radioecology and Environmental Radioactivity' (Part 2), Bergen, Norway, 15–20 June, pp. 129–132.

Covello V.T., 2011. Risk communication, radiation, and radiological emergencies: strategies, tools, and techniques. Health Physics, 101(5), 511–530.

Girard P, Heriard Dubreuil, G., 1996. Stress in accident and post-accident management at Chernobyl. *Journal of Radiological Protection*, 16(3), 167–180.

Heriard Dubreuil G, et al., 1999. Chernobyl post-accident management: The ETHOS project. *Health Physics*, 77(4), 361–372.

IAEA, 2000. Restoration of environments with radioactive residues. Proceedings of an International Symposium, Arlington, Virginia, USA, 29 November–3 December 1999. IAEA, Vienna.

ICRP, 1992. Radiological protection in biomedical research. ICRP Publication 62. *Annals of ICRP*, 22(3).

ICRP, 2006. The optimisation of radiological protection – Broadening the process. ICRP Publication 101b. *Annals of ICRP*, 36(3).

ICRP, 2007. The 2007 recommendations of the international commission on radiological protection. ICRP Publication 103. *Annals of ICRP*, 37(2–4).

ICRP, 2018. Ethical foundations of the system of radiological protection. ICRP Publication 138. *Annals of ICRP*, 47(1).

ICRP, 2020. Radiological protection of people and the environment in the event of a large nuclear accident: update of ICRP publications 109 and 111. ICRP Publication 146. *Annals of ICRP*, 49(4).

Kasperson R., Renn O., et al., 1988. The social amplification of risk: A conceptual framework. *Risk Analysis*, 8(2), 177–187.

Lochard J., 2013. Stakeholder engagement in regaining decent living conditions after Chernobyl. In: *Social and Ethical Aspects of Radiation Risk Management*, Oughton D., Hansson S.O. (Eds.), *Radioactivity in the Environment*, Vol. 9, Kidlington, Oxford, Elsevier, 2013, pp. 311–331.

Lochard J., Tabarre M., 1993. La robe et le nuage. Histoires de rayons X, de radioactivité et de radioprotection. Néo Edition. ISBN 978-2-914741-95-8.

Lochard J., et al., 2020. The post-nuclear accident co-expertise experience of the Suetsugi community in Fukushima Prefecture. *Radioprotection*, 55(3), 225–235. Available at: https://www.radioprotection.org/articles/radiopro/pdf/2020/05/radiopro200049.pdf

Maître M., Crouail P., Schneider T., et al., 2021. Living conditions and health status of populations living in territories impacted by nuclear accidents – Some lessons for developing health surveillance programmes. *Environment International*, 147, 106294 (article number).

Renn O., 1999. *A Model for an Analytic: Deliberative Process in Risk Management*, Vol. 33, NO. 18, 1999 / Environmental Science and Technology, pp. 3049–3055.

Renn O., 2008. *Risk Governance: Coping with Uncertainty in a Complex World*. Earthscan, London, Washington DC.

Ricœur P., 1991. *Lectures I: Autour du politique*. Seuil, Paris.

Ricœur P., 2017. *Philosophie, Ethique et Politique. Entretiens et Dialogues*. Seuil, Paris.

Schneider T, Lochard, J., 2021. Supporting societal and economic dynamic of recovery: Lessons from Chernobyl and Fukushima. In: Proceedings of the International Conference on Recovery after Nuclear Accident: Radiological Protection Lessons from Fukushima and Beyond. *Annals of ICRP*, 50(S1) (To be published).

Schneider T, Maître M, Lochard J, Charron S, et al., 2019. The role of radiological protection experts in stakeholder involvement in the recovery phase of post-nuclear accident situations: Some lessons from the Fukushima-Daïchi NPP accident. *Radioprotection*, 54(4), 259–270. Available at: https://www.radioprotection.org/articles/radiopro/full_html/2019/04/radiopro190069/radiopro190069.html

Slovic P., 2000. *The Perception of Risk*. Earthscan, London, Washington DC.

Takamura N, Orita M, Taira Y, Fukushima Y, Yamashita S., 2018. Recovery from nuclear disaster in Fukushima: Collaboration model. *Radiation Protection Dosimetry*, 182(1), 49–52.

UN, 1945. *Charter of the United Nations*. United Nations, San Francisco, CA.

USNRC, 2009. *Science and Decisions: Advancing Risk Assessment*. US Nation Academy of Sciences, Washington DC, USA.

Yasutaka T., et al., 2020. Dialogue, radiation measurements and other collaborative practices by experts and residents in the former evacuation areas of Fukushima: A case study in Yamakiya District, Kawamata Town. *Radioprotection*, 55(3), 215–224. Available at: https://doi.org/10.1051/radiopro/2020061

Zölzer F., 2016. Are the core values of the radiological protection system shared across cultures? *Annals of ICRP*, 45(S), 358–372.

Zölzer F., Zölzer N., 2020, February 25. Empathy as an ethical principle for environmental health. *Science of the Total Environment*, 705, 135922 (article number).

8 Citizen participation in post-accidental recovery

Radiation doses and welfare measurements

Liudmila Liutsko, Elisabeth Cardis, and Deborah Oughton

Introduction

There are many reasons for involving people affected by a nuclear accident in post-accident recovery. Involving people in the recovery process brings important knowledge and perspectives on accident mitigation. Their inclusion in actions can promote resilience, and their engagement can increase their trust in authorities and reduce psychological impacts (Oughton et al., 2021). There is also a fundamental ethical right for people to be involved in decisions that affect their lives (Hansson & Oughton, 2013; Liutsko et al. 2018). In practice, and in combination with developments on individual dosimeters and monitoring tools, citizen science provides an opportunity to increase public participation as well as promote transparency and communication.

Silvertown (2009) defines citizen scientist as a "volunteer who collects and/or processes data as a part of a scientific enquiry," but citizen science is not limited to mere data collection and processing. Citizens can also use their results as input to decision-making processes (Conrad & Hilchey, 2011). Involvement in scientific enquiries can also benefit citizens from an educational point of view (Dickinson et al., 2012; Newman et al., 2012), as it allows them to obtain new information and acquire new skills (Brown, Franken, Bonner, Dolezal, & Moross, 2016; Liutsko & Cardis, 2018; Naito et al., 2016).

Data collection in citizen science, including the so-called crowd-sourcing,[1] has limitations that need to be taken into account to avoid biases which may affect the interpretation of results. Wiggins and colleagues (Wiggins, Newman, Stevenson, & Crowston, 2011) found two main sources of errors in scientific research data gathered through public participation in data collection: protocols (not clear or poorly understood by citizens) and participants (people may not follow the same algorithms or methods as professionals). In the case of a nuclear emergency, part of this can be controlled by collecting information at multiple time points or by soliciting information through the apps before, during, and after the accident or intervention.

DOI: 10.4324/9780429318436-12

Recent developments in radiation protection and monitoring include dosimeters, applications, and social media sharing of data in the aftermath of the Fukushima Nuclear Power Plant accident (Liutsko & Cardis, 2018) with the *Safecast* (Brown et al., 2016) and *D-Shuttle* projects (Adachi et al., 2015). Citizen science also benefits from emerging new technologies, in particular mobile apps, that can provide useful tools to help educate citizens and provide support for data collection and management; reach more distant places and persons; and automate quality control (Newman et al., 2012). Citizens' involvement in dose measurements allows them not only to obtain information on doses they receive but also to make their own radiation protection decisions, adapting their behavior, for example by choosing to spend less time in the more contaminated areas or reducing or stopping consumption of food containing higher levels of radioactive contaminants. These aspects were found to reduce anxiety and improve the well-being of populations affected by the Fukushima nuclear power accident by adapting their own daily behavioral patterns (Naito et al., 2016; Murakami et al. 2018) and also to increase individual autonomy, liberty, and dignity—key ethical aspects in radiological protection (Oughton, 2016).

To conclude, both scientific research and public education can be advanced by citizen science, particularly when it is supported by organizational and professional association networks, open-access peer-reviewed journals, and cyber-infrastructure (Newman et al., 2012). In relation to nuclear accidents, these and other benefits of citizen science are explored in the SHAMISEN SINGS project (Liutsko et al., 2020; Liutsko, Sarukhan, et al., 2018; *SHAMISEN SINGS project*, 2018).

Objectives of the SHAMISEN SINGS project

The overarching goal of SHAMISEN SINGS was to enhance citizen participation in the aftermath of a radiation accident through the collection of data on dose measurements and on health and well-being indicators.

The specific objectives of the project, developed in the corresponding WPs (Figure 8.1), were the following:

- Interact with stakeholders (including citizens and experts) to assess their needs and interest in contributing to global dosimetry and health measurements (WP 1).
- Review existing apps related to: (1) citizen-based dose measurements and (2) health and well-being monitoring (including social and psychological issues of a radiation accident; WPs 2 and 3, respectively).
- Assess ethical challenges and implications of both the apps and citizen science activities by co-reflection between natural and social scientists, public, authorities, and other stakeholders as part of the concept and specification of apps and tools (WPs 1 and 4).

The SHAMISEN SINGS project reviewed and tested existing apps and questionnaires for monitoring dose and health and well-being. Based on this

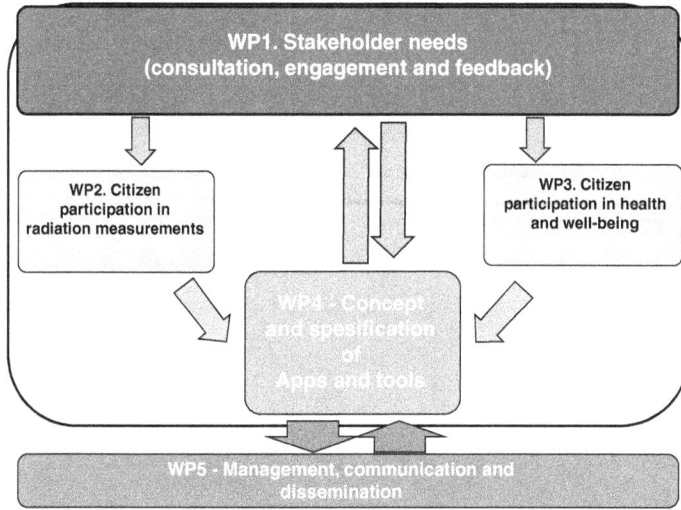

Figure 8.1 SHAMISEN SINGS project structure.
Source: *SHAMISEN SINGS project* (2018) and Liutsko, Sarukhan, et al. (2018).

review, criteria and examples of apps that could be used by citizens and for citizen science were drawn. These were discussed openly with relevant stakeholders during international and national events (conferences and workshops) during 2018 and 2019, and input from the stakeholders was taken into account in the recommendations.

The eventual outcome of the project was a set of recommendations regarding mobile apps (applications) for dose measurements and health indicators related to accidental or environmental radioactive exposure. Conceptualization and specification and development of apps that could be used by citizen science for dose measurements and health/well-being indicator after a nuclear accident (in emergencies and during long-term recovery) were performed by professionals—project participants and experts—in consultation with relevant stakeholders, including the general public. This chapter presents the results of various stakeholder interactions concerning the use of tools and apps by citizens for radiation monitoring.

The SHAMISEN SINGS WP1 survey on mobile apps and tools to measure external doses of radiation and health/well-being after nuclear accident

Recommendations on mobile apps (applications) for dose measurements and health indicators should reflect the needs and expectations of the general public and other relevant stakeholders. In order to evaluate the opinion of different stakeholder groups, a questionnaire was developed on *"Needs for apps (mobile applications) for dose measurements & health/well-being related to radiation exposure."*

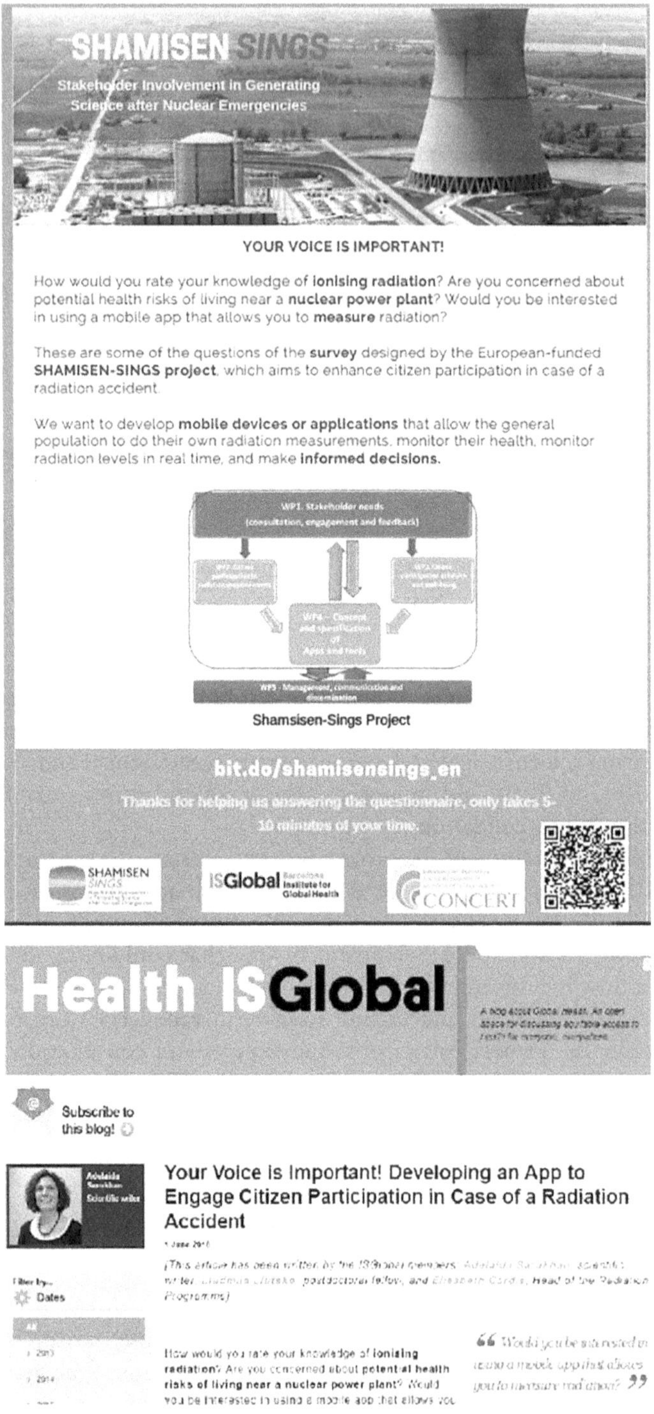

Figure 8.2 SHAMISEN SINGS survey leaflet (upper image, developed by Patricia Llobet, radiation group, ISGlobal) and a blog publication to engage general public in the survey (lower image, by Adelaida Sarukhan, ISGlobal).

This questionnaire was designed by partners and experts in the project from Spain, Italy, Norway, France, Ukraine, Belarus, and Japan. The original version of the questionnaire (in English) was translated into Spanish, French, Italian, Ukrainian, Russian, and Japanese. The link to the questionnaire was disseminated both electronically (via the ISGlobal blog's publication [Figure 8.2] and on the SHAMISEN SINGS website [*SHAMISEN SINGS project*, 2018]) and through leaflets with QR codes. No information permitting the identification of the participants in the questionnaire survey was collected.

Questionnaire scope and structure

The questionnaire contained four main blocks of information. *The first* collected general information about the survey participants: age group, sex, professional status, area of work or study, country and province/region of residence, level of education, and information about family nucleus (living with children or not, alone, etc.).

The second block aimed at obtaining information on the participants' self-assessment of their degree of knowledge and of concerns about ionizing radiation and sources. The participants were also asked whether they lived near an NPP.

The third block asked about the participant's potential interest in using mobile apps for measuring dose and/or assessing health and obtaining information/advice. Here, participants were also asked whether, in the case of using such an app, they would be willing to share their data collected through the app with other stakeholders (e.g., local authorities, doctors).

The fourth block was optional, targeting only persons who have already experienced a radiological or nuclear emergency. Questions were asked about their past experiences, such as access to information during emergency, application of radiation protection measures in daily life, and post-accident changes in behavior.

General survey results

The participants in the questionnaire survey (around 400, from 28 countries, but mainly from Belarus, Spain, Japan, Ukraine, France, Italy, Norway, and the UK) mostly had a high level of education (80% approximately) and only 11% did not know the meaning of the term *ionizing radiation*. The percentage of participants who were aware of existing mobile apps or device on dose measurements was lower (33%) than those who were aware of apps and devices to assess health (57%).

In terms of use of mobile apps, it is important to note differences in participants' perceptions and opinions on the use apps. Preliminary analysis of the English-speaking participants showed that 49% of participants considered that the use of mobile apps for dose measurements would be reassuring in case of an accident, 7% had no opinion, and 3% thought it would be stressful.

The rest of participants replied that it is "neutral" for them (neither beneficial nor harmful).

Among *difficulties* listed by participants who had previously used mobile apps (predominantly related to health and well-being), the following were the most frequently cited (quoted verbatim):

- Lack of appropriate instructions for use
- Difficult to login
- Too many parameters
- Does not provide much information
- Doubts about accuracy and reliability of data obtained with a mobile
- Use of difficult-to-understand medical terms
- Battery use (if the phone is in economy battery mode, the apps do not monitor)
- Technological barrier for elderly
- Excessive time needed to dedicate to data measurements
- Constant attention to the gadget on the phone to make repetitive measurements
- Very limited memory for synchronization when disconnected from the phone.

Suggestions for *improvement of* mobile apps included:

- Making them more interactive
- Use of easily understandable terms
- Conservation of battery life
- Clear description of the use of collected data: Will results/measurements be transferred to cloud servers (or not) and what happens with the collected data?
- Accurate calibration for dose assessment
- Improved measurement of physical activity; provide personalized information
- Ability to link with other apps to get the information that it needs (socio-demographical data, doses, health registers, etc.)
- Make data entry easier
- Allow the user to choose the parameters he/she wants to see
- Provide individual data feedback.

Data sharing and ethical aspects

An important benefit of citizen measurements is the possibility of sharing data at different levels including incorporating them into official environmental monitoring programs and/or having local authorities using them for decision-making processes. However, the sharing and exploitation of the data collected also raises a number of ethics and data protection and security issues. These aspects were discussed as part of a consensus workshop arranged by the project on issues related to the ethics of use and exploitation of mobile apps on dose measurements and relevant health indicators after a nuclear accident with the aim of informing and protecting health and well-being of the affected populations. Participants included the project partners (around 30%) and external experts from different countries (Norway, other EU countries, USA, Japan, Ukraine, and Belarus) and cultures and backgrounds (including one producer of mobile apps on dose measurements). The workshop drafted recommendations linked to the ethical aspects of app development (Oughton et al., 2019), which fed into the final SHAMISEN SINGS recommendations (Liutsko et al., 2020).

In addition to ethical issues linked to the sharing and use of data, the workshop highlighted the importance of user consent, especially the level of understanding that the participants have in providing that consent within apps. It was noted that there would be both practical and ethical differences between apps that provide information and those that advise on action. Both technical and ethical issues need to be addressed and made transparent in the experimental protocol for any citizen science project. This would include explaining links to organizations that might have interest in the results and their roles and functions. Given that current apps are at present largely driven by commercial actors, it was suggested that authorities take a more active role in the development and application of these tools, and it should be considered whether an international organization could take the lead on certification and data management. Finally, since the technology and the legal framework are likely to change, it is important that there is ongoing discussion focusing on the ethical implications of both technology and its use in citizen science projects (Oughton et al., 2019).

Survey results indicated that participants had different preferences concerning what information they were willing to share: (1) age (75%); (2) information on their current situation concerning exposure to radiation or to the consequences of an accident (71%); (3) location (68%); (4) health parameters (66%); (5) residence (59%); (6) physical activity (49%); (7) name/surname (28%); and (7) information of their family structure (22%). In general, 78% were willing to share their own information from apps either with professional stakeholders or for research purposes.

Technical aspects and measurements

Stakeholder feedback (from both the survey and group discussions) showed that both data collection and use of data (including by the citizens themselves) need to be accompanied by professional support. This could include professionals or intermediaries who can explain how to use these tools and interpret the data collected, as well as provide basic knowledge on radiation, units of measurements, and so on via direct or indirect interactions (i.e., chats). Concerning health apps, participants were less confused on their use since the majority of them had already used some kind of health mobile application and were therefore more familiar with them.

During meetings and discussions with citizens, other limitations on methods of dose measurements and radiation protection issues were mentioned. Since the official dose measurements are performed at the height of 1 meter, some citizens questioned their suitability for small children and wheelchair users and asked whether doses at lower heights should also be monitored. Children (together with pregnant women) are the most vulnerable population to radiation exposure and, thus, are considered to be at higher risk.

In general, it is not recommended to take measurements in highly contaminated areas, in order to avoid unnecessary exposure and possible negative consequences on health. Another issue to consider for citizen measurements with apps or devices in contaminated areas is the need for careful procedures to ensure that the recorded levels are not biased due to contamination of the device or phone during the measurement process. Personal protection is also important for those making their own measurements—recommendations include avoiding touching soils or other potentially contaminated materials and wearing gloves (Figure 8.3) and long sleeves to cover all open skin that could be in contact with radioactive particles.

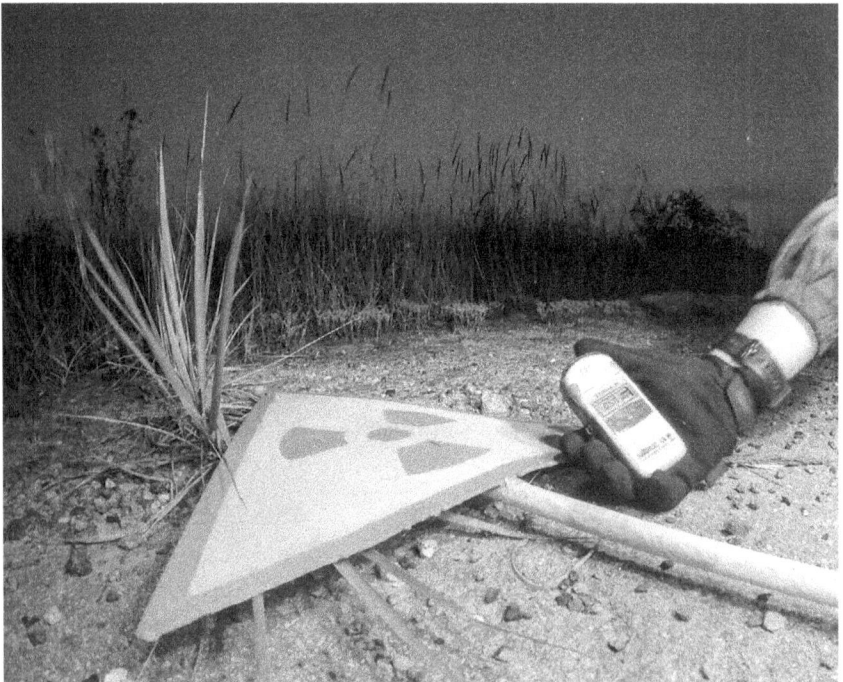

Figure 8.3 "Measuring radiation" by Gytizzz is licensed under CC BY-SA 2.0. Retrieved from https://ccsearch.creativecommons.org/photos/3a90e9f8-2c70-4910-bab3-055b2d2846dc
Note: Long sleeves and a plastic bag for a dosimeter are required for protection!

Benefits and challenges of citizen science in collection of dose and health/well-being data after a nuclear accident

The benefits of citizen scientists' participation in collecting data on radiation doses, especially for those who live in territories contaminated by past nuclear accidents (the consequences of which could last for decades or longer), include raising awareness, increasing knowledge, and developing a radiation protection culture among those who most need it. This is helpful not only for participants to increase their own protection, health, and well-being but also for all at the societal level, since the actions can also develop awareness and a radiation protection culture in the participants' family, social circles, and community. One person's behavior, knowledge, skills, and radiation protection culture can influence that of others—both contemporaries and future generations—and help those travelling to contaminated areas (Figure 8.4) for occupational or personal reasons, including tourism (e.g., Chernobyl tour[2]).

Due to technological advances, the quantity and variety of tools (including mobile apps) for dose measurements have increased rapidly in recent years. Some of them are simplified for general public use and include color codes to display levels of dose rates: *green* for normal and *red* for dangerous (Figure 8.5). Others are more technical. For them to be useful, however, easily understandable information should be provided or at least guidelines for members of the general public to be able to use them and interpret results obtained adequately clearly. It is also essential that the limitations of device and measurements be clearly provided, including specifying that the device or app cannot measure all types of radiation, info on what it actually measures, and guidelines for proper measurements (e.g., height of the device and duration of measurements).

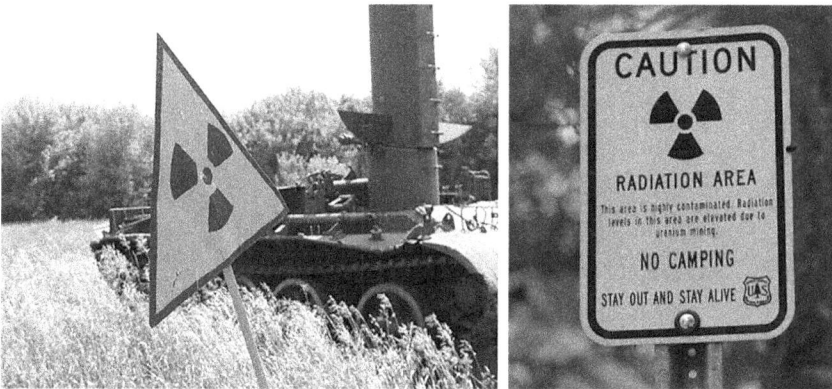

Figure 8.4 "Chernobyl and Pripyat" by Roman Harak and "Radiation Area" by caddymob are licensed under CC BY-NC-ND 2.0. Retrieved from https://ccsearch.creativecommons.org/photos/ec735e0a-7eb8-4102-bc63-cf731b6da3a4 (left) and https://ccsearch.creativecommons.org/photos/7f-d90db3-f661-4ce4-910f-4389212c3092 (right)

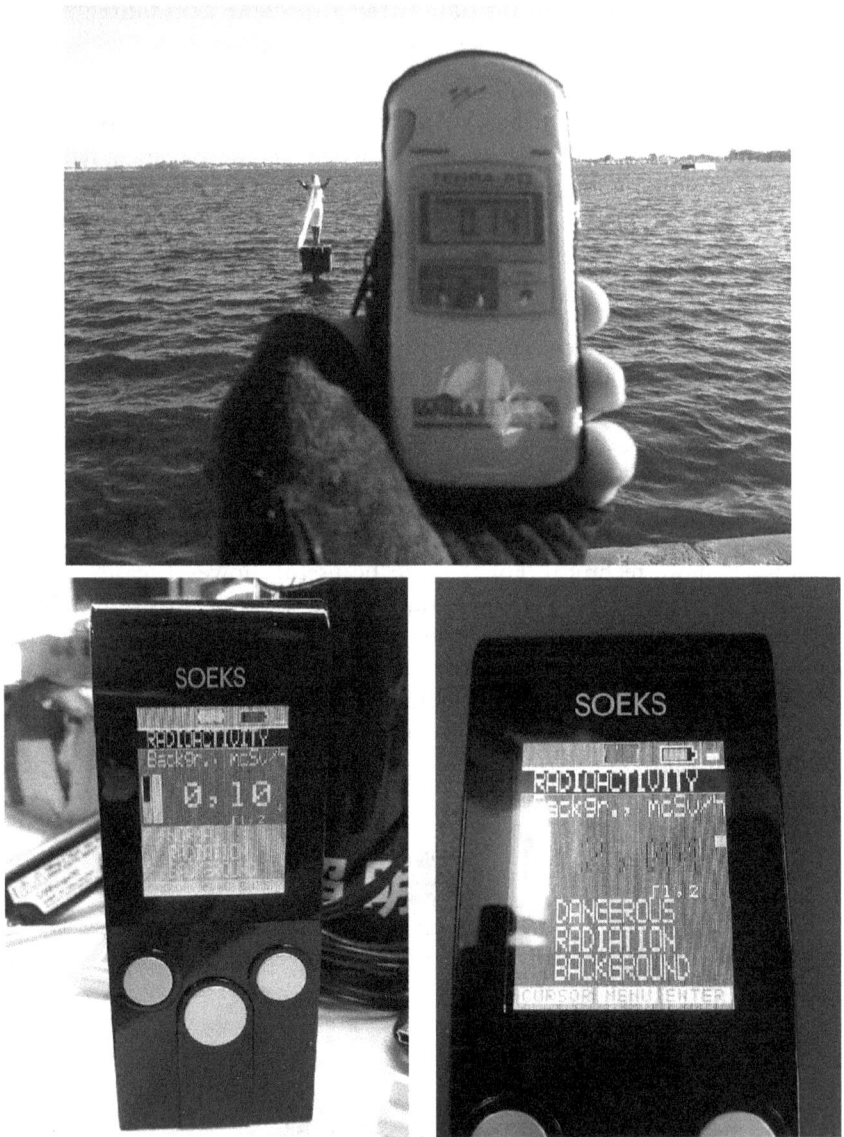

Figure 8.5 Radiation measurements tools for citizen.
Source: "10:13 16:00頃の中国地方上空" and "0.1uSv/h 2012/5/23 15:02 @ycam" by mhrs.jp is licensed under CC BY-NC 2.0 by mhrs.jp is licensed under CC BY-NC 2.0 and "0.14uSv/h 2013/11/27@matilda bay" by mhrs.jp is licensed under CC BY-NC 2.0. Retrieved from https://ccsearch.creativecommons.org/photos/4cb73c44-e756-4c3c-91f4-938cb14d8105 (on the left); https://ccsearch.creativecommons.org/photos/3473824e-a182-47ab-8683-2ce6a83d65ba (center) and https://ccsearch.creativecommons.org/photos/a7eece0e-ca2e-418b-934d-631c4152214e (on the right)

During the SHAMISEN SINGS project we reviewed the activities done in the Fukushima Prefecture that can be translated into apps on health and well-being of affected populations and prepared the general recommendations for app developers and relevant stakeholders and intended users (Goto et al., 2019; Liutsko et al., 2020). Such apps should consider not only the general aspects of any accident—stress due to changes that occurred, increased anxiety due to worries about health, economic issues related to these changes, and other negative consequences of the accident—but also those specific to nuclear accidents—such as diaries on daily behavior (that both help estimate personal exposure and reflect the status of health and well-being via data on quality of life and changes in behavioral traits and characteristics, including emotions, moods, and so on, post-nuclear accident). And from those thousands of health apps that already exist (Payne, Lister, West, & Bernhardt, 2015), a list of suitable ones could be selected with the capability to provide a complementary and more detailed examination of relevant aspects (e.g., quality of sleep and levels of anxiety or depression among the affected population).

Conclusions

Overall, the project concluded that data collected by individual citizens or in citizen science projects, if collected appropriately, can provide valuable information to authorities, complementing, in the cases of dose measurement apps, official environmental monitoring data. They can cover wider areas in more detail if many participants are involved, particularly in the early phases of an accident. Health and well-being data can provide a picture of how affected populations evaluate their health and well-being and of their needs after accident and how this evolves during the recovery period. This can help to better target and evaluate public health and their further psychological and social interventions that can also be performed with apps (Payne et al., 2015).

Moreover, if participants are willing to use both types of apps and to have their data on doses linked with those on health and well-being and geolocation, citizen science and other research projects could benefit from a potential database to study the relationship between dose and health. The results of such studies, in turn, would help characterize and better understand the harmful effects of radiation accidents on human health, leading to better interventions, and, in the case of possible future accidents, better preparation of preventive measures. In addition to the ethical benefits of public participation, there is also a need to consider the ethical implications of data use, and in particular who has access to results and how these might be used.

To sum up, citizen science is a growing field with the potential to make important contributions to the study of health consequences of radiation accidents and the definition and evaluation of interventions to mitigate them. The benefits are multiple; to the citizens themselves—engaging them in research on topics of concern (practical and theoretical) and educating them on these topics—to research scientists and to other relevant stakeholders, thus enhancing the potential for positive societal changes to emerge.

Acknowledgments

This work was conducted within the framework of the EC CONCERT–funded SHAMISEN SINGS project (Grant 662287, CONCERT, H2020). We acknowledge support from the Spanish Ministry of Science, Innovation and Universities through the "Centro de Excelencia Severo Ochoa 2019-2023" Program (CEX2018-000806-S), and support from the Generalitat de Catalunya through the CERCA Program.

Notes

1 Definition of crowdsourcing: https://dictionary.cambridge.org/es/diccionario/ingles/crowdsourcing
2 https://www.chernobyl-tour.com/english/

References

Adachi, N., Adamovitch, V., Adjovi, Y., Aida, K., Akamatsu, H., Akiyama, S., … Anzai, S. (2015). Measurement and comparison of individual external doses of high-school students living in Japan, France, Poland and Belarus—the "D-shuttle" project. *Journal of Radiological Protection*, 36(1), 49.

Brown, A., Franken, P., Bonner, S., Dolezal, N., & Moross, J. (2016). Safecast: Successful citizen-science for radiation measurement and communication after Fukushima. *Journal of Radiological Protection*, 36(2), S82.

Conrad, C. C., & Hilchey, K. G. (2011). A review of citizen science and community-based environmental monitoring: Issues and opportunities. *Environmental Monitoring and Assessment*, 176(1–4), 273–291.

Dickinson, J. L., Shirk, J., Bonter, D., Bonney, R., Crain, R. L., Martin, J., … Purcell, K. (2012). The current state of citizen science as a tool for ecological research and public engagement. *Frontiers in Ecology and the Environment*, 10(6), 291–297.

Goto, A., et al. (2019). D 9.137 – Preparation of core protocol for an APP to collect information on health and well-being. Retrieved from https://concert-h2020.eu/Document.ashx?dt=web&file=/Lists/Deliverables/Attachments/163/D9.137_Preparation%20of%20core%20protocol%20for%20an%20APP%20to%20collect%20information%20on%20health%20and%20well-being_approved04102019.pdf&guid=01b5ac77-b2ec-4cda-9c98-917dba396f0f

Hansson, S. O., and Oughton, D. 2013. Public participation—Potential and pitfalls, Chapter 18. *Radioactivity in the Environment*, 19, 333–345, ISBN 9780080450155. doi:10.1016/B978-0-08-045015-5.00018-6

Liutsko, L., & Cardis, E. (2018). P II–3–8 Benefits of participation citizen science in recovery programs (post-nuclear accidents). *Occupational Environmental Medicine*, 75(Suppl_1), A45–A46. doi:10.1136/oemed-2018-ISEEabstracts.115

Liutsko, L., Ohba, T., Cardis, E., Schneider, T., & Oughton, D. (2018). Socio-economic, historical and cultural background: Implications for behaviour after radiation accidents and better resilience. In F. Zölzer and G. Meskens (Eds.), *Environmental health risks: Ethical aspects* (pp. 28–42). Oxford: Routledge.

Liutsko, L., Sarukhan, A., Fattibene, P., Della Monaca, S., Charron, S., Barquinero, J. F., ... Goto, A. (2018). SHAMISEN SINGS project—stakeholders' involvement in generating science (radiation protection). *Arhiv za Higijenu Rada i Toksikologiju*, 69, 349–350.

Liutsko et al.; SHAMISEN SINGS Consortium★. (2020). *Mobile apps for monitoring radiation doses, health and welfare in the context of a nuclear or radiological accident: Guidelines and recommendations for users, developers and public authorities.* A pdf-printed booklet, available on-line: https://radiation.isglobal.org/shamisen-sings/booklets/

Murakami, M., Takebayashi, Y., Takeda, Y., Sato, A., Igarashi, Y., Sano, K., ... Tanigawa, K. (2018). Effect of radiological countermeasures on subjective well-being and radiation anxiety after the 2011 disaster: The Fukushima health management survey. *International Journal of Environmental Research and Public Health*, 15(1), 124. doi:10.3390/ijerph15010124

Naito, W., Uesaka, M., Yamada, C., Kurosawa, T., Yasutaka, T., & Ishii, H. (2016). Relationship between individual external doses, ambient dose rates and individuals' activity-patterns in affected areas in Fukushima following the Fukushima Daiichi nuclear power plant accident. *PLoS One*, 11(8), e0158879.

Newman, G., Wiggins, A., Crall, A., Graham, E., Newman, S., & Crowston, K. (2012). The future of citizen science: Emerging technologies and shifting paradigms. *Frontiers in Ecology and the Environment*, 10(6), 298–304.

Oughton, D. (2016). Societal and ethical aspects of the Fukushima accident. *Integrated Environmental Assessment and Management*, 12(4), 651–653.

Oughton, D., Ess, Ch., Tomkiv, Y., Liutsko, L., Cardis, E., Schneider, T., Fattibene, P., ... Sarukhan, A. (2019). Consensus workshop report on ethical aspects of radiation monitoring and health apps. Retrieved from https://www.researchgate.net/publication/341788401_Consensus_Workshop_Report_on_Ethical_Aspects_of_Radiation_Monitoring_and_Health_Apps. doi:10.13140/RG.2.2.20477.59363

Oughton, D., Liutsko, L., Midorikawae, S., Pirard, P., Schneider, T., & Tomkiv, Y. (2021). An ethical dimension to accident management and health surveillance. *Environment International*, 153, 106537. doi:10.1016/j.envint.2021.106537

Payne, H. E., Lister, C., West, J. H., & Bernhardt, J. M. (2015). Behavioral functionality of mobile apps in health interventions: A systematic review of the literature. *JMIR mHealth and uHealth*, 3(1), e20.

SHAMISEN SINGS project. (2018). Retrieved from http://radiation.isglobal.org/index.php/es/shamisen-sings-home

Silvertown, J. (2009). A new dawn for citizen science. *Trends in Ecology and Evolution*, 24(9), 467–471.

Wiggins, A., Newman, G., Stevenson, R. D., & Crowston, K. (2011, December). *Mechanisms for data quality and validation in citizen science.* In 2011 IEEE Seventh International Conference on e-Science Workshops (pp. 14–19). IEEE.

9 A new horizon in health research ethics

A view from the basis of radiological protection

Chieko Kurihara

Introduction

The theoretical framework of health research ethics has been expanding on the basis of established principles of biomedical ethics, mainly dealing with doctor–patient relationship toward a framework of broader view, incorporating environmental ethics or even corporate ethics, dealing with various topics considering populations or the ecosystem.

In 2018, the International Commission on Radiological Protection (ICRP) issued a publication of Ethical Foundations of the System of Radiological Protection (Publication 138).[1] They identified four core ethical values: beneficence/non-maleficence, prudence, justice, and dignity, along with procedural values: accountability, transparency, and inclusiveness. This set of core values seems to be a slight modification of the already established principles of biomedical ethics proposed by Beauchamp and Childress (1977).[2] However, this new set of values have the potential to be the basis for overviewing emerging issues in a new horizon in health research ethics.

First, this chapter articulates the evolution of health research ethics describing the characteristics of the established and the emerging frameworks. Second, it covers the evolution of radiological protection ethics—with the identification of core and procedural values. Finally, it shows practical examples of cases of health research that are related to radiological protection, presenting an analysis focused on the new values identified by the ICRP.

Evolution of health research ethics

Over the past half century, health research ethics have been evolving with expansion of framework, standing on the basis of established principles, acquiring broader view of recently emerging topics, and responding to the increasing demand from civil society. Table 9.1 shows the contrast between the framework with established principles ("established framework") and expanded framework with emerging topics ("emerging framework"). The established framework will never be replaced by the emerging framework. Instead, values identified in the emerging framework must be deemed as "additional" to those set in the established framework.

DOI: 10.4324/9780429318436-13

Table 9.1 Comparison between traditional and emerging models of health research ethics

	Established framework (framework with established principles)	Emerging framework (framework expanded with recently emerging topics, standing on the basis of the established framework)
Theoretical framework	• Doctor–patient relationship – Establishment of fundamental human rights - Expert's responsibility to protect individual's rights in deterministic circumstances (paternalism) • WMA's Declaration of Helsinki (DoH)	• Population/ecosystem interactions - Corporate social responsibility to protect the population/ecosystem in uncertain, stochastic circumstances - "Patient/ citizen-centeredness" • 2016 revision of CIOMS Guidelines • WMA's activities and revisions of DoH since 2000 • UNESCO 2005 Declaration on Bioethics
Dominant principles	• Beauchamp and Childress/ Belmont Report - Respect for autonomy/ person - Non-maleficence - Beneficence (These two were combined in the Belmont Report). - Justice	• Emmanuel et al., CIOMS 2016 - Social value - Community engagement/ collaborative partnership
Substantive requirement	- Informed consent - Privacy protection - Risk–benefit assessment/ management - Fairness of selection of research participants - Scientific validity: requirement of ethical justification - Study assessment and oversight by ethics committee	- Broad informed consent - Dynamic consent - Conflict of interest disclosure - Publication ethics (both positive and negative results should be published) - Social value: additional requirement of ethical justification, not only scientific validity - Avoid harm to humans as well as future generations, animals, ecosystem
Standard/ strategy to achieve justification	- Informed consent: information, conception, voluntariness - Safety assurance and compensation - Diversity of ethics committee members - Education, training	- Study registration in publicly accessible database - Sharing of individual patient data, respecting privacy - Shared responsibility, institutional governance, and citizen's oversight

(Continued)

	Established framework (framework with established principles)	Emerging framework (framework expanded with recently emerging topics, standing on the basis of the established framework)
Protection of vulnerability	- Protection of "categorized" vulnerable populations, for example, child, incompetent adult, pregnant woman, prisoner, poverty - Basically vulnerable populations should not be involved in risky research. Inclusion of vulnerable populations in the research must be justified ("Paternalistic")	- Protection of context-dependent vulnerability - Basically, vulnerable populations should be involved in research to generate knowledge for their specific health needs; Exclusion of vulnerable populations must be justified

Theoretical framework

The theoretical frameworks of health research ethics have been developed focusing on "a doctor-patient relationship," where a physician takes responsibility for the protection of the rights of an individual patient/research participant in deterministic circumstances, for example, in a small consultation room. This relationship is paternalistic because of the asymmetry of power and information. In 1947, the "Nuremberg Code" clarified the condition of acceptable human experimentation; the courts found Nazi physicians guilty of crimes against humanity during World War II. In 1948,[3] the United Nations Declaration of Human Rights established human dignity as the basis of freedom and equality of human beings. This framework of fundamental human rights was agreed in the International Covenant in 1966, and it prohibited human experimentation without informed consent.[4] Besides this international treaty, the World Medical Association (WMA) was established in 1947 and adopted Declaration of Geneva[5] in 1948 and the International Code of Medical Ethics[6] in 1949 to define the physician's obligations to prioritize patient care; then in 1964 they adopted the Declaration of Helsinki. This is the first set of internationally agreed ethical principles of medical research involving human subjects, and up to now it has been amended eight times.

In contrast, the expanded framework deals with recently emerging topics considering the "population/ecosystem interactions," where an organization has to take corporate social responsibility to protect not only individuals but also the population and/or ecosystem. Research organizations must adopt risk management procedures to minimize risks, based on probabilistic estimate. Patient advocacy groups and civil society have demanded more and more corporate governance of professional societies, research institutes, and, above all, industries. "The patient/citizen-centric model" is emerging, which promotes laypeople's commitment in the early phase of the research project. By this means, product development plan could become successful to respond the needs of these people and to gain social value of this product. The 2016 revision of the "International Ethical Guidelines for Health-related Research Involving Humans" by the "Council for International Organizations of Medical Sciences (CIOMS)," in collaboration with the World Health Organization (WHO), articulates this emerging framework.[7] CIOMS is a nongovernmental organization, jointly established in 1949 with the WHO and the United Nations Educational, Scientific and Cultural Organization (UNESCO). The CIOMS currently collaborates with more than 40 member academic societies, including WMA. Since their first guidelines in 1983, they have provided detailed commentaries on the principles in the Declaration of Helsinki, focusing on the context of the developing world. The 2016 revision has included the achievements of emancipated communities in the developing world to establish human rights in each jurisdiction. Before this development, the UNESCO Universal Declaration on Bioethics and Human Rights in 2005 provided the principles of bioethics to establish human rights, including people's equitable access to the development of medicine in a wider view of bioethics, not limited to research ethics.[8] Meanwhile, the WMA have issued various statements and social policy documents, as summarized in their Medical Ethics Manual.[9] Since the 2000 revision, the Declaration of Helsinki has come to include publication ethics, not only for protecting each research participant but also for disseminating credible research results. Besides this Declaration, the WMA has been engaged in global socioeconomic agendas, for example, medical issues in disaster situations, social determinant of health, and universal health coverage.

Dominant principles

The framework with established principles means the theory of bioethics with the set of three or four principles proposed by Beauchamp and Childress and the Belmont Report.[10] The principles dominant throughout the world are as follows: (1) Respect for autonomy/person (respect individual's decision-making and protect those with diminished capacity to make decisions); (2-1) non-maleficence; (2-2) beneficence ("do no harm" and maximize potential benefit; these two in Beauchamp and Childress were combined as "beneficence" in the Belmont Report); and (3) justice (fair distribution of risks and benefits of research; to avoid exploitation of vulnerable people exposed to research risks and providing benefit from research only to privileged people). This set of principles have been disseminated worldwide and considered as "principles of bioethics."

In the emerging framework, "social value" has been added to the above set of principles. Social value must never override the individual rights of a research participant. Social value means the importance of the knowledge that is expected to be generated as the result of a study, but it does not mean direct benefit to an individual study participant. For this reason, "community engagement" is a prerequisite to achieve social value, to affirm research questions responding to the health needs of the community and make research results available to them. It should be noted that "community engagement" does not allow community's permission substituting individual consent to research. This new set of principles, "social value" and "community engagement"/"collaborative partnership," which seem to be a paraphrasing or application of the "justice" principle, were proposed by Emmanuel et al,[11] adding to the above-mentioned established principles of bioethics. Then being incorporated in the 2016 revision of the CIOMS guideline, it comes to be acknowledged as an essential part of international framework of research ethics. This is one of the outcomes of long-lasting debates on HIV/AIDS perinatal transmission prevention placebo-controlled clinical trials that are sponsored by industrialized countries and hosted in developing countries. Several trials were conducted in developing countries to compare less effective and less costly therapy with a placebo, when there is any already established effective therapy, randomly assigning study participants to these therapeutic arms. Many have argued that such placebo-controlled trials exploit people living with HIV in poverty, generating research results mostly for people living with HIV in industrialized countries, because even if it was less costly it was still not affordable for people in the developing world.[12] Many others have argued that these trials are necessary to prove the effectiveness of less costly therapy and are better than nothing (placebo), in order to develop an affordable therapy for the people in a low resource-environment.[13] This debate has brought to light the need for achieving equitable, universal access to health, utilizing adequate human research as a stepping stone to this end.[14]

Substantive requirements

With the expansion of civil rights movement struggling with paternalistic medical society, the principles of bioethics have enabled to achieve patients' rights to informed consent. The principle of respect for autonomy/person requires "informed consent" of a research participant as well as privacy protection. The principle of beneficence requires the assessment and management of risks and benefits of research. The justice principle requires fairness in the selection of research participants. In this framework, scientific validity is the premise of ethical justifiability of the proposed research. This is because the research participant agreed to participate in the research with expectations of the results as explained in advance. The implementation of these principles must be assessed and monitored by a research ethics committee.

In the emerging framework, with the rapid development of information technology and globalization, interests of research community have been widely expanding to, for example, disaster situations (natural, manmade, war conflict); "big data" or whole-genome-sequencing analysis as well as biobank and health database[15]; and research using online/digital tools. In such situations, "data-driven research", including artificial intelligence (AI), to gather big amount of "real world data" or secondary use of data obtained in some previous research have come to be facilitated[16]. Thus, not only explicit informed consent to a specific research but also "broad informed consent" have come to be required. This does not mean a "blanket consent," but individual's consent with full understanding of various possibilities of future use of the data or material of this individual. Integrating both types of informed consent, "dynamic consent"[17] have been promoted, which enables a study participant (a donor of data/biomedical material) to make continuous decision to keep participation in new arising studies or withdrawal from them, by means of interactive information sharing, utilizing information technology. On the other hand, international community has continuously criticized against pharmaceutical company–funded research generating biased positive results to the sponsor company's drug. These positive results are often published, whereas the negative ones tend to remain unpublished, which leads to publication bias. Finally, the 2000 version of the Declaration of Helsinki has incorporated the ideas of publication ethics, with requirements of conflicts of interest disclosure, as well as publications of both positive and negative results. In this framework, "social value" is an "additional" requirement to scientific validity for the ethical justifiability of research. Additionally, with serious concern about the repeated pandemics and climate change, people come to require to avoid harm not only to the individual human being but also future generations as well as animals and plants in order to maintain a sustainable ecosystem.

Standard/strategy to achieve justification

So, what standards or strategies have been adopted in both frameworks? In the established framework, informed consent has been deemed valid by satisfying the three elements: "information" (giving sufficient information for candidates' decision-making); "conception" (sufficient understanding of the information provided); and "voluntariness" (avoiding undue influence, for example, inadequate excessive monetary incentive, or pressure from a superior to subordinate). Safety of each individual must be assured by describing risk minimization measures in the research protocol and qualified research team. Compensation for injury of a participant resulting from research has been deemed a moral obligation in terms of "compensatory justice."[18] To achieve these elements, oversight of an ethics committee with diversity of membership is required, including perspectives of committee members from a science educational background and those from a non-science educational background (e.g., expertise in humanities, study volunteers, or citizens); all genders; and external members who are not affiliated with the research institute. The education and training of individual researchers and ethics committee members are also required.

To avoid reporting bias and to expand usability of research results for evidence-based health care decision-making, international society agreed on the emerging ethical obligations of registration in the publicly available database of (1) clinical trial outline information at the beginning[19]; (2) results information at the completion; and (3) a plan for sharing with other researchers de-identified individual participant data (IPD) which are collected in the study.[20] This means that all the study information, including results and individual data to support the results, comes to be shared among responsible societies. As for the research governance framework, ethics committee oversight alone has come to be deemed insufficient; thus, the shared responsibility of a multidisciplinary team[21] and multidivisional institutional governance[22] have come to be required. Furthermore, with the development of information technology, citizen's oversight to increase transparency has become a recognized right.

Protection of vulnerability

Protecting vulnerable populations involved in the research has been one of the most critical issues of research ethics. Traditionally, vulnerable populations have been categorized into the following groups: children, incompetent adults, pregnant women, prisoners, people in poverty, people of lower status, institutionalized patients, and patients dependent on doctors. Basically, it was considered that vulnerable populations should not be involved in risky research. Therefore, rigorous justification is required for the "inclusion" of vulnerable populations. This is a somewhat "paternalistic" protection.

Recently, people have come to emphasize the protection of context-dependent vulnerability. This is because vulnerability will vary according to the context. Also, it has been argued that vulnerable populations should be involved in research to generate the knowledge needed for them. Therefore, justification is required for the "exclusion" of vulnerable populations. Even if these reversed theories of protecting the vulnerable have become dominant, you must never sacrifice or compromise on the safety of these vulnerable people in order to achieve meaningful research results. Consequently, you have to not only achieve the "respect of individual's rights" (not involve unwilling vulnerable people in risky research) bur also focus on "social value" to promote research that generates knowledge which is valuable for them (CIOMS 2016).

Evolution of radiological protection ethics

Establishment of radiological protection ethics

In the next part, this analysis shows that the set of core and procedural values proposed by the ICRP Publication 138 could be the basis of the above-mentioned emerging framework of health research ethics. In the ICRP Publication 109 (2009), Clarke and Valentin clarified the correlation between the main theories of ethics and the development of the radiological protection system.[23] This is not in an official statement by the ICRP but in an invited article. Later their analysis was introduced in the ANNEX of the Publication 138, which can be summarized as follows:

- **Early recommendations** (1928–1950s): Responding to the discovery of X-ray, their recommendations have focused on avoiding deterministic effects in medical occupational exposure. The theoretical ethical basis has been Aristotelian "***virtue ethics***," where human beings keep their "inner sense" of moral orientation.
- **Intermediate recommendations** (1960s–1970s): Next stage was for managing stochastic effects, providing a balance between risks and benefits in society. ICRP's principles of justification and optimization and the "as low as reasonably achievable" (ALARA) principle have been developed on the basis of "***consequence ethics***" ("***utilitarianism ethics***").
- **Present recommendations** (1980s to present): Limitation principle entails applying dose limit to protect the rights of the individual in an equitable manner; thus, "limits should be set to avoid sacrificing one person for the sake of others." This idea is directly linked to "***deontological ethics***" ("***duty ethics***").

Then, in 2018, Publication 138 presented ICRP's official analysis on their evolution of recommendations and its ethical basis, paraphrasing in terms of the core ethical values: beneficence/non-maleficence, prudence, justice, and dignity. It also explains in the ANNEX that there are three main levels of ethical theories classified as

> ***meta-ethics*** (discussing the general meaning of ideas such as "virtue," "good," or "right"), ***normative ethics*** (discussing how one should act, and which values and norms should be followed), and ***applied ethics*** (discussing specific issues, e.g. in medicine or engineering, based on ethical theories or principles).

The above three ethical theories in Clerk's analysis are all in the scope of "normative ethics." Based on this historical analysis, the ICRP clarified on the four core ethical values as the foundation of radiological protection system and proposed the same in Publication 138. This set of values is similar to the principle of bioethics, which founded the basis of "applied ethics" in this field. Similarly, this proposal of the set of core ethical values established the basis of "applied ethics" in the field of radiological protection. This can be called "radiological protection ethics," equivalent terminology to "medical ethics," "environmental ethics," and so on, beyond the scope of normative ethics (Figure 9.1).[24]

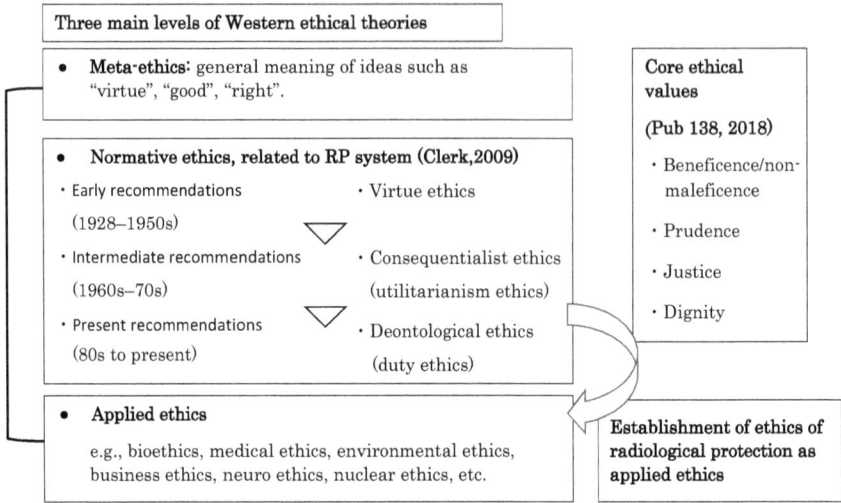

Figure 9.1 Challenges of ICRP: To the next step.

Several prominent publications have already called for applied ethics in this field[25] that discusses practical issues. However, what is important is that the ICRP has established their own core ethical values. So what is the difference between normative ethics and applied ethics? Normative ethics discusses "norms"—recommending what you should do or should not do, integrated into regulations, guidelines, recommendations, or policies. Meanwhile, applied ethics deals with any kind of actual problems we face—and various types of outcomes can be generated: sometimes regulations or on other occasions some actions in the real world to implement respectful values. Applied ethics has been established in various disciplines. The most prominent is bioethics, which can deal with any topic that is related to "life."[26] Medical ethics and environmental ethics are subcategories of bioethics. Research ethics, engineering ethics, and corporate or business ethics are also prominent. "Radiological protection ethics" could also be a subcategory within bioethics as it mainly deals with the issue of life. However, it also contains some considerations in the area of corporate/business ethics or engineering ethics as it demands an ethical code of conduct of industries.

Comparison between established and emerging value sets

Along with these core values, ICRP have expanded their view with the procedural values of accountability, transparency, and inclusiveness. When we compare the ethical principles of health research and the ethical values of ICRP, there is interesting concurrence (Table 9.2). The similarities between the principles of bioethics and the ICRP core values are not coincidental but intentional. This is because many of the Task Group (TG) members discussed

Table 9.2 Concurrence of a set of principles/values between health research ethics and ICRP's radiological protection system

Health research ethics principles	Established framework	Emerging framework
	Beauchamp and Childress/ Belmont Report (principles of bioethics) Combined in Belmont Report - Respect for autonomy/person - Non-maleficence - Beneficence - Justice	Emmanuel et al., CIOMS 2016 - Social value (additional to the left, never override individual's rights) - Community engagement
ICRP ethical values	**Core values** - Beneficence/non-maleficence - **Prudence** - Justice - **Dignity**	**Procedural values** - Accountability - Transparency - Inclusiveness

these bioethics principles (you can find all the presentations of the TG on the website: http://www.icrp.org/page.asp?id=237). Meanwhile, the similarity between the principles in the emerging framework of health research ethics and the procedural values of ICRP is unintentional. TG members did not discuss Emanuel's proposal of a new set of principles or CIOMS 2016 revision. So why were these similar value sets raised coincidentally?

In the established framework, the value set is to be implemented by an individual, or a group of experts, as may be necessary for each research project or radiological protection program. The set of values which has appeared in the emerging framework dealing with "population/ecosystem interactions" is to be implemented by various groups of people. Early inclusiveness (participation) of stakeholders in a fair and effective manner is essential to maintain transparency and accountability. It is not only ethical behavior but also successful achievement and availability of the outcome that are demanded. This means that experts take a greater deal of responsibility than ever before to meet the larger demands of society. Simultaneously, stakeholders are taking shared responsibility for decision-making throughout the duration of the project, right from the beginning to the end. Furthermore, implementation of the value set is not completed within one particular project.

Another point for consideration—why do differences exist between the set of values in the established framework and ICRP's core ethical values? These two value sets are similar, but the following two points of modification, using traditionally established classic notions (prudence, dignity), reflect the characteristics of the expanding view in the emerging framework:

1   To include "prudence" in addition to the established value set
    Publication 138 described "prudence" as "the ability to make informed and carefully considered choices without full knowledge of the scope and

consequences of actions." This is rooted in Western philosophies (Plato and Aristotle), as well as in non-Western theories (Confucius[27,28] and others[29]). This value is related to the modernized "precautionary principle"[30] of making a decision in the situation of uncertainty to avoid unpredictable risks. This should not just be deemed as never taking risks. "It describes the way in which decisions are made, and not solely the outcome of those decisions" (Publication 138).

The principles of bioethics have been used as a useful analytical tool to solve ethical dilemmas, clarifying values to be respected as objectives of an action, and it does not include the internal mechanism of the subject of an action. Meanwhile, the ICRP value set incorporates "prudence"—the decision mechanism of the subject of an action. The traditional value set was articulated with the premise of the unarticulated existence of a reasonable person who can make a rational judgment and balance these sometimes conflicting values. This means that the decision-making mechanism exists in a different dimension from the value set. However, in the society of the emerging framework, related stakeholders make the decision collectively. This inevitably incorporates an additional value of "prudence"—which represents the decision-making mechanism.

2   To replace "respect for autonomy/person" with dignity

"Dignity" is the fundamental attribute of a human being, which means "every individual deserves unconditional respect, irrespective of personal attributes or circumstances such as age, sex, health, disability, social condition, ethnic origin, religion, etc." This is a superordinate concept of autonomy. For this reason, both persons with autonomy (self-determination capacity) and those with diminished autonomy equally deserve human rights, derived from human dignity. The Belmont report states that a person with diminished autonomy deserves to be given additional protection. Furthermore, dignity has been attributed not only to living individuals (with special attention to humans in the process of dying) but also to the deceased, a human embryo or fetus (thus abortion and discarding of a human embryo can be permitted under some conditions), nonhuman species, or even to nature.[31] The ICRP is neutral as to whether it is anthropocentric (the ecosystem has to be preserved for the sake of human beings who deserve dignity) or biocentric (the ecosystem is valuable enough in itself to be preserved). The ICRP has not stated that nonhuman species and nature deserve dignity. But at least they expand the scope of protection to fauna and flora.[32] This fits with the emerging model of ethics that expands the moral obligations of protection not only to individuals but also to populations and the ecosystem.

Now we can find an interesting contrast between "prudence" and "dignity." Prudence represents wisdom in a self-governing capacity, which is defined by Kantian philosophy as a reason of human dignity.[33] "Prudence" has been deemed as the highest virtue of a human being. Historically, this virtue has been deemed to be exerted by an expert with professional autonomy. Meanwhile, human dignity is an attribute of every kind of person—with special emphasis on the most vulnerable and disadvantaged. This contrast articulates the picture in the emerging model, where experts and lay people share decision-making and actions collaboratively. In this framework, beyond the utilitarian theory, solidarity and empathy[34] among all the related stakeholders would promote "social value," without sacrificing the dignity of the individual and the community.

Examples: view from procedural values

Finally, this analysis poses some practical issues to be further explored, focusing on the values newly identified by the ICRP (prudence, dignity, and the three procedural values) and discussing four case examples of health research ethics related to radiological protection. All of these are issues the author has faced frequently in day-to-day practice but are summarized using general descriptions.

Example 1: Diagnostic radiology research

Issues in the established framework

ICRP Publication 62 (published in 1992[35]) provides a unique project evaluation tool for the radiological protection of participants involved in clinical research, showing the categories of risk and corresponding levels of benefit (Table 9.3). The International Atomic Energy Agency (IAEA) Safety Standards (2014[36]) state that research cannot be justified without considering this publication along with the Declaration of Helsinki and the CIOMS.

Importantly, a study in excess of 10 mSv could be justified if it generates "substantial societal benefit," which is explained as "usually directly related to the saving of life or the prevention or mitigation of serious disease." However, in some of the PET (positron emission tomography)/CT (computed tomography) diagnostic imaging studies involving healthy volunteers, the total effective dose of multiple scans in one study protocol may exceed 10 mSv. Sometimes these volunteers participate in similar studies repeatedly, although many of the study protocols exclude volunteers who have participated in another study within the past several months. Publication 62 recommends avoiding repeated participations, but there are no established measures to avoid it.

Table 9.3 Categories of risk and corresponding levels of benefit, shown in the
ICRP Publication 62[a]

Level of risk	Risk category[b]	Corresponding effective dose (adults, mSv)	Level of societal benefit[c]
Trivial	I (~10^{-6})	< 0.1	Minor
Minor to	IIa (~10^{-5})	0.1–1	Intermediate to
intermediate	IIb (~10^{-4})	1–10	moderate
Moderate	III (~10^{-3} or more)	>10^{d}	Substantial

a Slightly modified from the original table in the ICRP Publication 62. The following notes
are quoted or abbreviated from the main text or note under this table in this publication.
b "The total detriment from the exposure; namely the sum of the probability of fatal cancers,
the weighted probability of non-fatal cancers and the probability over all succeeding generations of serious hereditary disease resulting from the dose." Children detriment per unit
dose is two to three times larger; for people aged 50 years or over it is about 1/5th to 1/10th
of that for younger adults; for those suffering from serious diseases radiation-induced risk
will be even lower.
c The level of social benefit corresponding to the risk category I: "only to increase knowledge"; IIa: Increases in knowledge leading to health benefit"; IIb: "more directly aimed at
the cure or prevention of disease"; III: "usually directly related to the saving of life or the
prevention or mitigation of serious disease" or in case the "potential benefit is directly to
the participant."
d "To be kept below deterministic thresholds except for therapeutic experiments."

Some believe that research involving a healthy volunteer with radiation
exceeding 10 mSv would be difficult to get approval for (as ICRP demands
"substantial societal benefit"), and ICRP suggests it should only "be kept
below deterministic thresholds (which is far beyond 10 mSv) except for therapeutic experiments." Meanwhile, the U.S. Food and Drug Administration
(FDA) legally defines the following range of radioactive drug administration
to be deemed "safe": 3/5 rem (≒30/50 mSv) single/annual dose for the whole
body; active blood-forming organs; lens of the eye; gonads; or otherwise
5/15 rem (≒50/150 mSv) single/annual dose for other organs.[37] Any clinical
study over this range requires the approval of the FDA before starting. As
such, there is a difference between FDA and ICRP in the risk categorization.
Moreover, there is no internationally agreed recommendation by ICRP to
control what is the acceptable annual accumulated dose for the healthy volunteers for whom there is no direct therapeutic benefit.

Strategies in the emerging framework

The "societal benefit" described in Publication 62 is similar to—but not
identical with—the above-mentioned "social value" in the emerging framework. "Social value" is not limited to the medical knowledge used to treat
"serious" cases, but it can be applied to any kind of health-related outcomes
that are meaningful for society. In addition, it calls for a fair, equitable availability of the research result for the people who need it.

Publication 62 recommends that a radiological protection expert(s) should be included in the research group, as well as in the ethics committees. In addition, in the emerging framework, explicit discussion is needed involving research participant populations (*inclusiveness*). Healthy volunteers, as well as patients of cognitive impairment or mental disorder, both moderate or severe, would often participate in these kinds of studies. This population, along with families or relatives and general citizens, should be involved in the discussion on what is the "substantial societal benefit" to justify radiation risks over 10 mSv. In addition, *transparency* to register these studies in public databases is required for the sake of citizens' oversight.

Example 2: Radiation therapy research

Issues in the established framework

The ethics of radiation therapy is especially critical when involving a pregnant woman or those of childbearing age. ICRP Publication 84[38] provides meaningful information for the protection of both woman and fetus—according to the volume of radiation dose and target region and associated risks to the fetus. It states that "pregnant women should not be involved in biomedical research projects involving radiation exposure unless the pregnancy itself is central to the research—and only if alternative techniques involving less risk cannot be used." This text was originally written in Publication 62, and it also states that the proposed benefit should substantially exceed the possible detriment; informed consent must be obtained from the pregnant patient and "it would usually be appropriate to seek the same from the father." This policy should be carefully implemented considering the following points:

1 Routine exclusion of women of pregnant or childbearing age may deprive them of the opportunity to access radiation therapy research with potential direct benefit, and it causes a lack of evidence of potential risks and benefits to these populations.
2 Such a routine exclusion policy may also cause the researcher to be unwilling to engage in difficult consultation with the women, whether or not to participate in research with potential benefit of anticancer effect, but high or absolute possibility of termination of pregnancy or loss of reproductivity.
3 It may be better to obtain consent both from a pregnant woman and a father of the fetus; however, we should be careful with some specific situations where the interests of the woman and father conflict. We should be especially cautious in a society where women's rights have not been well recognized, contrary to internationally established norms to assure their rights (Declaration of Human Rights).

Strategies in the emerging framework

To explore the strategies in the emerging framework, CIOMS 2016 version states that "Women must be included in health-related research unless a good scientific reason justifies their exclusion." This contrasts with the theory in the established framework which tends to exclude women from health-related research because of their childbearing potential. It also recommends the promotion of research "to obtain knowledge relevant to the health needs of pregnant and breastfeeding woman" because of their "distinctive physiologies and health needs." It also states that:

> Only the informed consent of the woman herself should be required for her research participation. Since some societies lack respect for women's autonomy, in no case must the permission of another person replace the requirement of individual informed consent by the woman.

This represents the recent trend of protecting the vulnerable population (not only women but also children or incapable adults, etc.), requiring justification of exclusion, rather than justification of inclusion. Also, the decision-making process should be facilitated, for the best interest and benefit of the vulnerable research participant, which may be supported by the surrounding people, with careful consideration of possible conflicting interests. Publication 84 promotes collaborative decision-making among the patient, husband (or spouse), or other appropriate person(s) and also with medical team members (e.g., radiologists, surgeons, obstetricians, pharmacologists, and others such as psychologists or member of the clergy), considering various interdisciplinary medical elements as well as legal, ethical, and moral issues. This kind of shared decision-making model should be *prudently* facilitated in the newly emerging societal circumstances of health research ethics. In any case, it must never override the intrinsic decision rights that are private to the woman participating in any research, in terms of respecting her *dignity*.

Example 3: Research in radiation disasters

Issues in the established framework

In the case of radiation disaster, the rapid initiation of monitoring, survey, or research involving the affected population is essential. It is imperative to collect accurate data of radiation dose at the onset of the event and during the succeeding early phase. Without such initial data, the complete picture of the disaster may be lost, or biased results may be generated.

Not only government, public, or private institutions but also individual or groups of citizens may conduct surveys in disaster situations. This includes radiation measurement and behavioral recordings of citizens, as well as emergency radiation workers, from whom urine and/or blood sample may be collected. In some cases, the researcher may be faced with a situation where it is difficult to get approval from the ethics committee and the consent from each of the research participants as well as doing it in time so as not to lose essential information. On the other hand, affected citizens may start to gather their own data utilizing mobile devices and a social network system, not as a part of the research study, but as self-help activity.

Japanese people have bitter experiences of "guinea pig claims." In Hiroshima, Nagasaki, shortly after the atomic bombing, a U.S.-oriented survey followed survivors' natural history but did not provide care. There were also similar claims in the case of the Fukushima nuclear accident. The residents expressed suspicion toward surveys of local government or academic researchers, which took place without providing relevant care for them. It caused researchers' attitude to pretend to be providing "support" and not conducting a "survey."[39] Some of such projects were conducted without ethical review approval. In other cases, they have failed to obtain critically important study data, because of taking style of support, not of research. Consequently, these studies may lose ethical justifiability and/or compromise "scientific validity." Therefore, "social value" is also lost, which is an essential component of ethical justifiability.

Strategies in the emerging framework

ICRP's Publication 146[40] entitled: "Radiological protection of people and the environment in the event of a large nuclear accident: Update of ICRP Publication 109 and 111" describes the whole picture of disaster response, focusing especially on the protection of people and the environment, respecting the established core and ethical values. It also specifies the prerequisites to monitoring—survey and epidemiological study—which should be incorporated in the disaster response both in the emergency and recovery situations.

The 2016 CIOMS guidelines provide important suggestions for how research in a disaster situation should be carried out giving due consideration to the following key points before embarking on the research project:

- Research should form an integral part of disaster response.
- Research can be met with great skepticism or even hostility; researchers must be equipped to negotiate these pressures in fragile political and social situations.
- An acute situation may *require an* accelerated ethical review to ensure that necessary studies can begin as soon as possible without compromising ethical requirements.
- "Generic protocol approval," which can be prepared at the vulnerable disaster areas (earthquake, tsunami, as well as nuclear plant areas), in advance of the event, to make possible "accelerated (abbreviated) ethical review" at the time of emergency.

Expanding these suggestions, we should aim for building consensus on the following:

1   **Develop a theoretical framework to define the boundary between "disaster response" and "research"**: We need this theoretical framework as a premise for ethical conduct of research in disaster situations—as it is defined in the Belmont Report on the boundary between "practice" and "research." This would help to clarify the activities that do not require ethical approval and the others that need it. Also, many of the disaster response activities will later transition into a research study; thus, we should clarify the mechanism to get ethical approval at this transitional phase.

2   **Citizen-oriented research**: Citizens themselves may start to measure their radiation dose for the protection of family or small units of community and may start to communicate with other communities. This is a valuable step in self-help activities to develop radiation protection culture to overcome a disaster situation.[41] Sometimes, such accumulation of data may generate valuable scientific knowledge that deserves to be published in academic meetings or journals. Specialists and other relevant stakeholders may be invited to collaborate from the initial or middle stage in this process. Such activity may not fit into the central dogma of prior ethical approval. This needs the above-mentioned clarification of boundaries between "disaster response" and "research." This process would lead to *prudent* decision-making of residents collaborating with experts, respecting the *dignity* of individuals and communities. Also, valuable scientific knowledge would be disseminated to wider communities and future generations (*transparency and accountability*).

3   **Waiver of individual consent, assuring dignity and social value**: "Generic protocol review" and "abbreviated additional review" strategy mentioned above could incorporate the justification theory of gathering citizens' data without obtaining individual consent. Thus, what kind of research is needed for the people in some disaster situations and under what conditions waiver of consent could be justified should be thoroughly discussed as a part of preparedness. In this process, community-oriented consensus development is a prerequisite (*transparency accountability* and, above all, *inclusiveness*). Based on such deliberation, some kinds of essential research may be justified for the abbreviation of some of the traditional procedures. In any case, the dignity and rights of the individual and the community must not be overridden (*dignity*).

4   **Alternative method of ethical review**: As a possible alternative system of ethical review, the "international electronic ethics review system" may provide some solution. The electronic review system by Medicines Sans Frontier (MSF, Doctors Without Borders) shows one example.[42] It provides faster and high-quality review for research performed by MSF in emergency situations, constructing a panel from the international pool of experts of ethics.

Example 4: Radiation epidemiology

Issues in the established framework

Long-term epidemiological surveys of radiation effects are extremely important, because the radiological protection systems have long relied on the scientific evidence generated from these epidemiological studies. There are two prominent types of difficulties: (1) continuous following of life history including accurate information about the cause of death and (2) whether or not to disclose incidental (unsolicited) or secondary findings and research results to the participants and/or related community and how the right of the participants to adequate treatment should be assured.

The first issue is becoming increasingly difficult because of the strengthening of personal data protection. CIOMS provided the first guidelines for epidemiological research in 1991, and the Declaration of Helsinki expanded their scope in 2000 to individual-identifiable data or human sample. Moreover, the legal protection of personal data has become stricter worldwide. In this situation, a long-term large-scale prospective epidemiological survey to follow radiation workers or residents of high-radiation-dose areas must require the full informed consent of participants—except in some types of legally defined surveys where individual consent may be waived. In some regions, "broad informed consent" (one-time consent for broad, roughly categorized future research, given sufficient information) and/or "information disclosure and opt-out" (information of each research is widely disclosed offering an individual the opportunity of the option to be excluded from the study) may be justified by laws and/or regulations. However, for obtaining accurate information of the cause of death from a local government or hospital, explicit consent in advance of the person concerned and/or consent of the responsible representative of the deceased would be needed. If it is only a matter of gathering de-identified statistical data, then it may not pose such difficulties, but sometimes it is not enough because studies that aim to estimate the correlation between exposure and outcome need to maintain a link between individual and outcome information.

Issue two (2) can be classified into two categories of issues of information disclosure: (i) incidental (unsolicited) or secondary findings and (ii) research results.

i Incidental (unsolicited) or secondary findings means any health-related information found unintentionally in the course of research procedures. Sometimes it is a directly research-related one (e.g., higher radiation dose than expected, found through experimental method of analysis) or otherwise it may not be assumed to be related to the research (e.g., some specific serious disease found by blood test, which generally is not related radiation effect);

ii Research results and intentional findings, proven by research, may impact each study participant, the parent population, and the related community. Sometimes it leads to the development or improvement of health
policy and otherwise it may cause discrimination or stigmatization
against specific populations.

For this reason, it has been regarded to be the researcher's ethical obligation
to have clear and adequate communication with participants and the related
community about (i) incidental findings and (ii) research results in terms of:

- Meaningfulness of returning incidental findings/research results to an
  individual, considering analytical validity, clinical significance, and
  actionability.
- Respect both for the "right to know" and "right not to know" of study
  participants. (Researcher should provide options to participants to be or
  not to be informed.)
- Publication of research results in a scientifically valid manner and considering the positive and negative impacts on both the participants and
  the related community.
- To provide necessary care and/or health and social policy for the individual and/or the related community responding to these findings.

Strategies in the emerging framework

The recent strengthening of personal data protection has evoked the idea
of "ethical obligation of participating in research." This argument comes
from the recognition that the social security system (including the health
care system) has been developed based on research evidence—and all bene-
ficiaries should take responsibility for participating in enterprises to develop
evidence. This may be seen as a "trick" to override an individual's right
to refuse to participate in research. Therefore, fundamental agreement between the research community and society is required—with an assurance
of protecting *dignity* and safety, and with a shared perspective of "social
value." This also must incorporate adequate and sufficient measures to prevent discrimination or stigmatization against the persons or populations
who may be affected by the study results.[43] And above all, benefit as the result of research must be fairly shared among the community. Only the process with *transparency*, *accountability*, and fair *inclusiveness* with profound
maturity of solidarity and empathy could lead to *prudent* decision-making
as a society.

In this process, citizens are involved in each step of the planning of basic
policy of the community—as well as in each research protocol design; research implementation and data analysis; manuscript development and results
dissemination; and implementation of research results in the society, which

include logistics and socioeconomic strategies. Research participants would be able to be engaged in all or some parts of these processes, according to their ability and motivation.[44] And of course their participation has to be accepted through an adequate informed-consent acquisition process (*dignity*). Through this process, consensus could be reached for returning an incidental finding to an individual and publicizing the results widely to the community and throughout the world (*transparency*), strengthening strategies of benefit sharing to assure global health.

Conclusion

The theoretical framework of health research ethics has developed and evolved in the form of norms of international agreements since the end of World War II. In this process, the expansion from the established framework to an emerging framework reflects the transition from paternalism that focuses on the doctor–patient relationship to a citizen-centric initiative that focuses on corporate social responsibility being integrated with environmental ethics or corporate/business ethics. The theoretical framework of radiological protection system has evolved over the past hundred years, leading to clarification of its core and procedural values in the past decade, with the establishment of applied ethics of this field. This value set is in concurrence with the emerging framework of health research ethics, both fortuitously and inevitably. This value framework has great potential to view and analyze recent challenges in a new horizon; integrating all the disciplinaries of health research ethics, environmental ethics, and radiation protection ethics. In all processes, we must assure the protection of the dignity and human rights of research participants as well as the achievement of social value to protect global health for all, along with sustainability of ecosystem.

Acknowledgments

I deeply appreciate Professor Kimberly E. Applegate, MD, PhD, Department of Radiology, University of Kentucky School of Medicine (retired), United States Professor Sandor Kerpel-Fronius, MD, PhD, Department of Pharmacology and Pharmacotherapy, Semmelweis University, Hungary Professor Dirceu Greco, M.D., Ph.D., Professor Emeritus, Infectious Diseases and Bioethics, Federal University of Minas Gerais, Brazil and Professor Tom Beauchamp, PhD, Professor Emeritus, Georgetown University, United States, who provided significantly important comments and revisions on this manuscript.

The author is a member of ICRP TG 94 for Publication 138 and TG 109 for Ethics in Radiological Protection for Medical Diagnosis and Treatment. However, this chapter only describes the author's personal view (except for the texts with explicit references).

Notes

1 International Commission on Radiological Protection. Ethical foundations of the system of radiological protection. ICRP Publication 138, *Ann. ICRP*, 2018; 47(1).
2 Beauchamp TL, Childress JF. *Principles of Biomedical Ethics*, 3rd ed. Oxford University Press, Inc.; 1977.
3 United Nations, 1948. The Universal Declaration of Human Rights [On line]. Adopted 10 December 1948.
4 United Nations, 1966. International Convent on Civil and Political Rights. Adopted and opened for signature, ratification and accession by General Assembly resolution 2200A (XXI) of 16 December 1966, entry into force March 1976.
5 The World Medical Association. The Declaration of Geneva. First adopted in September 1948, last amended in October 2017. Available from: https://www.wma.net/policies-post/wma-declaration-of-geneva/
6 The World Medical Association. The International Code of Medical Ethics. Adopted in October 1949, last amended in October 2006. Available from: https://www.wma.net/policies-post/wma-international-code-of-medical-ethics/
7 Council for International Organizations of Medical Sciences. *International Ethical Guidelines for Health-Related Research Involving Humans*. 2016.
8 United Nations Educational, Scientific and Cultural Organization. *Universal Declaration on Bioethics and Human Rights*. 19 October 2005.
9 World Medical Association. *Medical Ethics Manual*, 3rd ed. 2015. Available from: https://www.wma.net/what-we-do/education/medical-ethics-manual/
10 DHEW. National Commission for the Protection of Human Subjects of Biomedical and Behavioral Research. The Belmont Report. Department of Health, Education and Welfare. 1979. Available from: http://videocast.nih.gov/pdf/ohrp_belmont_report.pdf (PDF) (DHEW pub. no. (OS) 78-0012). Washington, DC: United States Government Printing Office.
11 Emanuel EJ, et al., eds. *The Oxford Textbook of Clinical Research Ethics*. New York: Oxford University Press; 2008, pp. 123–135.
12 Lurie P, Wolfe SM. Unethical trials of interventions to reduce perinatal transmission of the human immunodeficiency virus in developing countries. *N. Engl. J. Med.*, 1997; 337: 853–856.
13 Varmus H, Satcher D. Ethical complexities of conducting research in developing countries. *N. Eng. J. Med.*, 1997 Oct 2; 337(14): 1003–1005.
14 Greco DB. Emancipation in the struggle for equality in research involving human volunteers. *Rev. bioét (Impr.)*. 2013; 21(1): 19–30.
15 World Medical Association. WMA Declaration of Taipei on ethical considerations regarding health databases and biobanks. Adopted by the 53rd WMA General Assembly, Washington, DC, USA, October 2002 and revised by the 67th WMA General Assembly, Taipei, Taiwan, October 2016.
16 Kurihara C, Baroutsou V, Becker S, Brun J, Franke-Bray B, Carlesi R, Chan A, Collia LF, Kleist P, Laranjeira LF, Matsuyama K, Naseem S, Schenk J, Silva H and Kerpel-Fronius S. Linking the Declarations of Helsinki and of Taipei: Critical Challenges of Future- Oriented Research Ethics. *Front. Pharmacol.* 2020. 11: 579714. doi: 10.3389/fphar.2020.579714
17 Kaye J, Whitley EA, Lund D, Morrison M, Teare H, Melham K. Dynamic consent: a patient interface for twenty-first century research networks. *Eur J Hum Genet.* 2015; 23(2):141–6.
18 Levine RJ. *Ethics and Regulation of Clinical Research*, 2nd ed. Yale University Press; 1988.
19 De Angelis C, Drazen JM, Frizelle FA, Haug C, Hoey J, Horton R, Kotzin S, Laine C, Marusic A, Overbeke AJ, Schroeder TV, Sox HC, van der Weyden

MB. Clinical trial registration: A statement from the International Committee of Medical Journal Editors. *NEJM*, 2004; 351(12): 1250–1251.

20 Taichman DB, Backus J, Baethge C, Bauchner H, de Leeuw PW, Drazen JM, Fletcher J, Frizelle FA, Groves T, Haileamlak A, James A, Laine C, Peiperl L, Pinborg A, Sahni P, Wu S. Sharing clinical trial data: A proposal from the International Committee of Medical Journal Editors. *PLoS Med.*, 2016; 13(1): e1001950. doi:10.1371/journal.pmed.1001950.

21 Kerpel-Fronius S, Becker S, Barrett J, Brun J, Carlesi R, Chan A, Collia LF, Dubois DJ, Kleist P, Koski G, Kurihara C, Laranjeira LF, Schenk J, Silva H. The shared ethical responsibility of medically and non-medically qualified experts in human drug development teams. *Front Pharmacol.*, 2018 Sep 3; 9: 843. doi:10.3389/fphar.2018.00843.eCollection2018

22 Federman DD, Hanna KE, Rodriguez LL, eds. Committee on Assessing the System for Protecting Human Research Participants, Institute of Medicine of the National Academies. In *Responsible Research: A Systems Approach to Protecting Research Participants*. Washington, DC: National Academies Press; 2002.

23 Clarke RH, Valentin J. The history of ICRP and the evolution of its policies. In ICRP Publication 109. 2009.

24 Kurihara C. On the ICRP Publication 138 "Ethical Foundation of Radiological Protection System": Developing process and its outline. *Jpn. J. Health Phys.*, 2019; 54(1): 19–29.

25 Oughton D. Ethical values in radiological protection. *Radiat. Prot. Dosim.*, 1996; 28: 203–208.

26 Kimura R. Bioethics as a prescription for civic action: The Japanese interpretation. *J. Med. Phil.*, 1987; 12(3): 267–277.

27 Tsai DFC. Ancient Chinese medical ethics and the four principles of biomedical ethics. *J. Med. Ethics*, 1999; 25: 315–321.

28 Kurihara C, Cho K, Toohey RE. Core ethical values of radiological protection applied to Fukushima case: Reflecting common morality and cultural diversities. *J. Radiol. Prot.*, 2016; 36: 991–1003.

29 Zölzer F. A cross-cultural approach to radiation ethics. In: Oughton D, Hansson SO (Eds.), *Social and Ethical Aspects of Radiation Risk Management*. Elsevier Science, 2013: pp. 53–70.

30 United Nations Educational, Scientific and Cultural Organization (UNESCO). The Precautionary Principle. March, 2005.

31 Huber W. Rights of nature or dignity of nature? *Ann. Soc. Christian Ethics*, 1991; 11: 43–60.

32 ICRP. Protection of the environment under different exposure situations. ICRP Publication 124. *Ann. ICRP*, 2014a; 43(1).

33 Kant I. *Groundwork of the Metaphysic of Morals*. 1785.

34 Malone J, Zolzer F, Meskens G, Skourou C. *Ethics for Radiation Protection in Medicine*. 2019; CRC Press.

35 ICRP. Radiological protection in biomedical research. ICRP Publication 62. *Ann. ICRP*, 1992; 22(3).

36 IAEA, FAO, ILO, et al. Radiation protection and safety of radiation sources: International basic safety standards. IAEA Safety Standards Series No. GSR Part 3. International Atomic Energy Agency, Vienna.

37 Code of Federal Regulations Title 21: Food and Drugs, Volume 5, Part 361: Prescription drugs for human use generally recognized as safe and effective and not misbranded: Drugs used in research: Sec. 361. 1: Radioactive drugs for certain research uses (40 FR 31308, July 25, 1975).

38 ICRP. Pregnancy and medical radiation. ICRP Publication 84. *Ann. ICRP*, 2000; 30(1).

39 Kurihara C. Ethics and radiation protection in biomedical research in the post-Fukushima era: Up to date. 14th International Congress of the International Radiation Protection 9–13 May 2016, Cape Town International Convention Centre, South Africa. Page 244 to 252 of the Proceedings. Available from: http://www.irpa.net/docs/IRPA14%20Proceedings%20Volume%201.pdf

40 ICRP. Radiological protection of people and the environment in the event of a large nuclear accident: update of ICRP Publications 109 and 111. ICRP Publication 146. Ann. ICRP, 2020; 49(4).

41 Lochard J, Schieber C. The evolution of radiological risk management: An overview. *J. Radiol. Prot.*, 2000: 20: 101–110.

42 Schopper D, Upshur R, Matthys F, Singh JA, Bandewar SS, Ahmad A, van Dongen E. Research ethics review in humanitarian contexts: the experience of the independent ethics review board of Médecins Sans Frontières. *PLoS Med.*, 2009 Jul; 6(7): e1000115. doi:10.1371/journal.pmed.1000115. Epub 2009 Jul 28.

43 Kurihara C, Inoue T. Ethics, regulations and clinical development of precision medicine: Activating with molecular imaging. In: Inoue T, David Y, Huan G (Eds.), *Personalized Pathway-Activated Systems Imaging in Oncology: Principal and Instrument.* Springer; 2017: pp. 105–126.

44 Alberta SPOR SUPPORT Unit. Patient engagement in health research: A how-to guide for researchers. May 2018 (Version 8.0).

Part 4

Research ethics for environmental health

10 Roles for ethical and social values in environmental health research

Kevin C. Elliott

Introduction

This chapter seeks to broaden conceptualizations of research ethics in environmental health. It is typical for curricula in research ethics or the responsible conduct of research (RCR) to focus on a relatively narrow array of issues such as data management, authorship, mentoring, animal welfare, and respect for human research subjects (Shamoo and Resnik 2015). In some cases, the curricula might extend a bit more broadly, to encompass concerns about how scientific and technological advances impact society (e.g., Shrader-Frechette 1994). In this chapter, I will argue that research ethics for environmental health should be conceptualized even more broadly so that it includes decisions embedded in the cognitive aspects of doing research, such as the formulation of questions and hypotheses, the development of models, the analysis and interpretation of data, and the communication of scientific results.

To establish the need for this broader conception of research ethics, the chapter reviews recent literature from the philosophy of science on the roles that ethical and social values play in scientific research. It shows that environmental health researchers are forced to make a wide variety of value judgments. Some scholars have suggested that scientists should adopt a "value-free ideal," according to which they avoid appealing to ethical or social values when making these judgments. I argue that this approach is ethically problematic for environmental health researchers. Instead, I suggest that they adopt a "value-management ideal" that focuses on three principles for handling value judgments in a responsible fashion: transparency, representativeness, and engagement. The chapter places special emphasis on transparency, suggesting a number of strategies that can be used for promoting transparency about value judgments in ways that meet people's informational needs. These strategies involve not only environmental health researchers but also a range of other actors and institutions, including scholars from the humanities and social sciences, science journalists, and government agencies. Thus, the chapter concludes that addressing the full range of ethical issues associated with environmental health research will require system-level thinking and multifaceted approaches.

DOI: 10.4324/9780429318436-15

A broad conception of research ethics for environmental health

In order to understand the need for a broadened conception of research ethics for environmental health, it is helpful to refer to a set of distinctions developed by Nancy Tuana. Within the overarching field of research ethics, she distinguishes between three types of ethical issues: procedural ethics, extrinsic ethics, and intrinsic ethics (Tuana 2010). She places issues related to data management, proper credit for authorship, responsible mentoring, management of financial conflicts of interest, and proper treatment of human and animal research subjects in the category of *procedural ethics*. Her category of *extrinsic ethics* focuses on efforts to apply science and technology in ways that fairly distribute benefits and burdens and that promote social welfare. Finally, Tuana defines *intrinsic ethics* as "ethical issues that are internal to or embedded in the production of a given inquiry or mode of analysis" (Tuana 2010, 480).

It is easy to miss the significance of intrinsic ethics because it involves subtle choices that scientists may not even recognize to be ethically significant. For example, Kristen Intemann (2015) has highlighted a number of ways in which climate modelers make decisions that might not initially seem to be ethically significant but that can have important consequences for society. For example, she points out that the decision to tune a model to make it particularly good at predicting some phenomena (e.g., the distribution of precipitation across a particular region) can make it less successful at predicting other phenomena (e.g., extreme weather events). Similarly, given limited resources, the development of models that are good at describing gradual climatic changes may conflict with the goal of developing models that are good at predicting worst-case scenarios. Deciding what kinds of models are most important to develop is an ethically and socially significant question. To take a slightly different example, Intemann also points out that many integrated assessment models (IAMs) are designed to report information about the overall economic costs and benefits to society of taking particular responses to climate change. She notes that it is an ethically significant choice when models are designed to provide this sort of aggregated information for society as a whole rather than disaggregated information about how economic costs and benefits will be distributed across particular groups, such as those who are already disadvantaged in various ways.

The sorts of intrinsic ethical issues highlighted by Tuana and Intemann constitute a particularly rich domain of research ethics that deserves much more exploration. Recent work in the philosophy of science provides a good starting point for exploring this topic, because philosophers of science have been exploring how the choices made by scientists throughout the research process can end up serving some social and ethical values over others. The next section of this chapter provides an introduction to this scholarship on "science and values" in order to show how it can help clarify the intrinsic ethical issues that arise in environmental health research.

Introduction to values and value judgments in research

The philosophical literature on science and values has flourished in recent years (see, for example, Longino 1990; Douglas 2009, 2016; Elliott 2017; Elliott and Steel 2017; Fernández Pinto and Hicks 2019). Values are often defined as qualities or states of affairs that are desirable or worthy of pursuit. There is room for philosophical disagreement about precisely what makes these qualities desirable (Brown 2018), but for practical purposes there tends to be widespread agreement about which things count as values. Initially, philosophers of science tended to focus on epistemic values, which are qualities like explanatory power or predictive power that apply to scientific theories or hypotheses and that provide reasons for thinking they are true or reliable (see, for example, Steel 2010; Douglas 2013). More recent discussions of values in science have placed greater attention on the ways in which scientific choices can promote ethical and social values like public health, environmental sustainability, economic development, fairness, opportunity, and so on (see, for example, Douglas 2016; Elliott 2017).

Values are relevant to scientific inquiry because scientists are forced to make value judgments throughout the course of their work. Value judgments are choices that are not constrained by logic and available evidence. These judgments include choices about what topics to study; what questions to ask; what background assumptions to adopt; how to develop and tune models; how to design studies; how to collect, analyze, and interpret data; how to categorize phenomena; how to weigh different forms of evidence; how much evidence to demand before drawing conclusions; how to frame and describe findings; and how to use and apply scientific results. In most cases, scientists make these decisions without consciously appealing to particular values. Nevertheless, when working on applied topics like environmental health, these decisions still end up being value-laden, in the sense that they end up supporting some values over others depending on how they are made (Elliott 2017; Ward 2021).

One might respond in various ways to this realization that scientists make value-laden judgments throughout the course of their research. One approach has been to insist that scientists should try as much as possible not to consider social or ethical values, at least when engaging in "core" aspects of scientific reasoning like assessing theories and hypotheses (see, for example, Betz 2013; Hudson 2016). Proponents of this approach recognize that social and ethical values have a legitimate role to play in some aspects of science, such as deciding to prohibit research practices that are unethical. They also acknowledge that scientists cannot completely avoid being influenced in various ways by their personal values. Nevertheless, they contend that when evaluating the evidence for their theories and hypotheses, scientists should at least strive to minimize the influences of social and ethical values on their reasoning. Frequently called the "value-free ideal," the goal of this approach is to prevent values from harming the objectivity of research.

In recent years, however, the value-free ideal has come under significant criticism (see, for example, Douglas 2016). One of the most important reasons for rejecting the value-free ideal is that it seems to violate the ethical responsibilities of scientists to consider the consequences of their actions, and especially to avoid negligently causing harm to others. As Heather Douglas (2017) has emphasized, scientists can have a significant impact on society when they draw conclusions about practical topics like medicine, nutrition, energy, agriculture, economics, and the environment. Depending on the consequences of being wrong, she argues that scientists should consider how much evidence to demand before making pronouncements that could have a significant effect on those around them. Douglas's argument appears to apply particularly well to environmental health scientists because they frequently make claims that can have significant consequences for society. For example, environmental health researchers are often asked by policymakers to discuss the likely consequences of climate change or the dose levels at which industrial chemicals are likely to cause harm or the range of health effects associated with pesticides. Thus, it makes sense for them to follow Douglas's advice and to consider the consequences of being wrong when deciding how much evidence to demand before drawing conclusions (see, for example, Douglas 2009; Elliott and Richards 2017).

Decisions about how much evidence to demand before drawing conclusions are not the only socially important choices that environmental health researchers make. As discussed in the previous section, their decisions about how to design and tune climate models influence which questions they are able to answer with precision (Intemann 2015). When designing toxicology studies, their choices about how long to let the studies run, which animal models to use, and which biological endpoints to measure can influence whether the studies tend to exonerate the chemicals under investigation or find them to be harmful (Elliott 2014, 2016). Similarly, their decisions about how to weigh many different kinds of evidence (sometimes including computer modeling as well as in vitro, animal, and epidemiological studies) can determine whether they conclude that potential hazards are a cause for concern or not. Environmental health researchers also have to make choices about how to interpret ambiguous data, such as evidence for low-dose toxic effects that are not observed at higher doses; some researchers take these apparent effects to be legitimate, whereas other researchers argue that they are likely spurious (see Vandenberg et al. 2019). Similarly, researchers have to make judgments about whether specific biological effects caused by environmental hazards (e.g., changes in enzyme levels or organ weights) are likely to translate into overall adverse effects for organisms or populations (Elliott 2011). Thus, scientific research is like a "tapestry" composed of a host of value judgments; scientists are constantly making choices that are not settled by the available evidence but that can have impacts on society (Elliott 2017).

Given that scientific research in fields like environmental health involves an endless array of value judgments that cannot be settled by the available evidence but that can have significant impacts on society, it would be eth-ically irresponsible to tell scientists to ignore the consequences of the judg-ments they make. Instead, it is important for scientists to develop systems for making these judgments responsibly. Proponents of the value-free ideal are correct to think that it would be problematic if scientists idiosyncrati-cally accepted hypotheses solely because they fit with their preferred personal or political perspectives. Nevertheless, it would be equally problematic for scientists to make all the value-laden judgments associated with their re-search with no consideration for the social consequences of making them one way rather than another. In order to handle all the intrinsic ethical issues involved in making the judgments associated with their research, scientists working in the field of environmental health need a "value-management ideal" to help them operate responsibly. The next section suggests what a value-management ideal might look like.

A value–management ideal for environmental health research

Deciding how to handle the value-laden judgments involved in scientific research is a hot topic in contemporary philosophy of science. A number of proposals have been put forward, and it is likely that a combination of them will ultimately be needed (see Resnik and Elliott 2019). Most of these pro-posals are related to three general principles for managing values in science responsibly: transparency, representativeness, and engagement (Elliott 2018).

Transparency

First, transparency involves making the value judgments involved in envi-ronmental health research as clear as possible for those who need to make decisions based on that research. Transparency is important because it can help people to use scientific research for making thoughtful decisions even when the research has been influenced by value judgments. In contrast, failing to make value judgments transparent can sabotage people's ability to make good decisions. For example, consider the case of climate mode-ling. As governments make plans for adapting to rising sea levels, chang-ing precipitation patterns, and increased temperatures, they will rely on climate scientists to help them understand the conditions they could be facing in the future. As we have seen, however, climate scientists have to make a host of decisions when developing their models. Some decisions might make them more likely to overestimate the potential incidence of particular threats, while other decisions might make them more likely to underestimate them. If those receiving information from climate modelers do not understand how the information they receive could be influenced by these judgments, they are likely to make poor decisions that do not ac-cord with their own values.

Researchers tend to be aware of the importance of transparency, and they have taken a variety of steps to promote it. For example, scientists are trained to acknowledge major value judgments associated with their research in the "Discussion" sections of their journal articles, and they typically acknowledge important judgments in media interviews as well. Similarly, many journals now require the authors of journal articles to disclose financial conflicts of interest (COIs) so readers can be on the lookout for ways in which those COIs might have influenced important judgments (Elliott 2008). Government agencies that deal with environmental health issues, such as the U.S. Environmental Protection Agency (EPA), also take a number of steps to help clarify important value judgments. One of these steps is to develop scientific advisory boards and panels that scrutinize the research performed for regulatory purposes and identify important judgments associated with it. Another step is to produce reports that synthesize available information and communicate about its strengths and weaknesses in ways that are meaningful for both policymakers and members of the public. International bodies like the Intergovernmental Panel on Climate Change (IPCC) have also taken extensive steps to try to quantify the uncertainties and limitations associated with their predictions and to communicate about those uncertainties in effective ways (Havstad and Brown 2017).

Unfortunately, environmental health researchers—and scientists in general—are still a long way from achieving complete transparency about value judgments. Part of the problem, as Justin Biddle and Eric Winsberg (2010) have argued, is that value judgments are often hidden in the "nooks and crannies" of scientific research; thus, it is often difficult for scientists to recognize all the ways in which their work could have been influenced by important judgments. Another problem is that those who want to receive information about value judgments typically vary a great deal. For example, some members of society are particularly risk-averse, and they are likely to want a great deal of information about the value judgments associated with assessing environmental threats. Other people are likely to find all this information to be distracting and confusing. Similarly, some people might not need much assistance to be able to understand important value judgments, whereas others might need a great deal of explanation (Elliott 2020). In a field like environmental health, where the findings are relevant to non-specialists, it is especially important to find ways to communicate about value judgments in ways that are meaningful to the wide range of people who want to make use of this information (Elliott and Resnik 2019).

Another important problem is that even though transparency can provide a warning to those who do not agree with the way important judgments in research have been handled, in many cases this still leaves those who disagree with the judgments unable to make use of the research that was performed. For example, Andrew Schroeder (2019) has made a distinction between fixed and user-assessable value choices. In the case of user-assessable value choices, it is possible for the recipients of scientific information to go back and reanalyze the results to determine how they would differ if alternative judgments had been made. However, many value choices are what Schroeder terms "fixed"; in these cases, it is difficult or impossible to determine what alternative results would have been obtained if different judgments had been made. A particularly extreme version of this problem occurs with what James Robert Brown (2010) calls "one shot science." In cases of one-shot science, only a few big studies (and perhaps only one) are performed on a particular topic. If those studies are designed in ways that serve some values over others (e.g., tending to underestimate or overestimate the chemical's toxicity), those who hold differing values are left unable to determine what results would have been obtained using a different study design.

Representativeness

Because of one-shot science and other challenges, such as the difficulty of achieving full transparency about value judgments, it is also important to strive for what I have called "representativeness" about value judgments. The basic idea is that judgments in science should be made in ways that accord with or "represent" major ethical and social priorities (Elliott 2017). Thus, if society tends to place greater priority on protecting public health than on promoting the economic growth of the chemical industry, toxicology studies should be designed so that they tend to overestimate rather than underestimate the toxicity of the chemicals under investigation. To the extent that representativeness in environmental health research can be achieved, society can be provided with information that is well-designed for meeting societal priorities.

A weakness of my previous work on the topic of representativeness, however, is that it does not specify exactly how to determine whether particular judgments have been made in ways that are adequately representative (Brown 2018; Kourany 2018). Contemporary societies are characterized by a great deal of polarization, which means that it is difficult to arrive at ethical principles or social priorities that are universally shared. Thus, arriving at an adequate account of representativeness becomes difficult, although various approaches have been proposed.

One strategy is to develop an approach for engaging in ethical reasoning about which values should inform value judgments. The basic idea of this approach is that as long as our values are well-justified from an ethical perspective, it does not matter if some people disagree with them; we can still justifiably use them to guide value judgments in science. For example, Matt Brown (2020) appeals to a Deweyan ethical framework for reasoning about value judgments. According to the Deweyan framework, ethical inquiry is grounded in problem-solving; thus, scientists can determine how to handle difficult value judgments by looking at the problem situation that scientific inquiry is designed to solve and exploring which judgments are best for addressing that problematic situation. In her book, *Philosophy of Science after*

Feminism, Janet Kourany (2010) also argued for using ethical principles to manage value judgments in science.

To the extent that these approaches call for ethical reflection on the judgments that permeate environmental health research, they are valuable. As a stand-alone solution for managing values in science, however, they are incomplete. In most difficult cases, there is simply too much uncertainty involved in ethical reasoning for it to be the sole solution to addressing value judgments in science. Reasonable people can disagree about how best to solve problematic situations, and most ethics codes and guidelines do not address all the detailed judgments that scientists need to make (Resnik and Elliott 2019).

Andrew Schroeder (2020; 2021) suggests responding to ethical disagreement about value judgments using a political approach. In other words, he argues that value judgments in science should be made in ways that fit democratic values, that is, the values of the public and their political representatives. This proposal coheres well with my principle of representativeness, but Schroeder has developed it with greater care and detail. He does not specify a particular approach for identifying democratic values, but he suggests various possibilities. One option would be to engage in a procedure, such as an exercise in deliberative democracy or a referendum. Another option would be for political philosophers to examine empirical evidence about the public's values and, after removing values that are clearly ethically problematic or ill-founded, clarify the core values present among the public.

Although Schroeder's proposal is attractive in many respects, one might worry that it would be difficult to implement. Stephen John (2015) has suggested a slightly different and much simpler approach. He focuses on value judgments involving the amount of evidence required for drawing conclusions, and he argues that scientists should make them in a uniform way that always involves a high standard of evidence. This approach might not initially appear to be very representative of the array of values present among members of the public, but John points out a sense in which it is representative. Specifically, by requiring a uniformly high standard of evidence, it enables all members of society to trust the results that scientists report, because they know that whatever their own standards of evidence might be, the results are likely to meet them. As noted previously, John focuses specifically on judgments involved in deciding how much evidence to demand before drawing conclusions, but his approach could perhaps be adapted to other value judgments as well. His core idea is that standardized approaches to handling value judgments could make science trustworthy for all members of society (see also Wilholt 2013).

Schroeder's and John's proposals provide valuable options for those seeking to address value judgments in environmental health research, but they still face weaknesses. For one thing, despite Schroeder's promising suggestions, it is still not an easy matter to decide what the democratic values are in a society, especially when there is a great deal of polarization. Schroeder (2021) acknowledges that one could employ multiple (perhaps conflicting) democratic values in some cases if there were significant disagreements within society, but deciding when to employ more than one value and what that value or values should be is a complex matter. Second, whether one employed democratic values (as Schroeder suggests) or uniform values (as John suggests), there would still be many people in society who hold different, minority values. Thus, while those minority groups might acknowledge that science based on the democratic or uniform values is legitimate for making large-scale political decisions, it would still be reasonable for them to draw different conclusions when making decisions that apply primarily to themselves and not to the rest of the society. To take a concrete example, one could imagine a government agency like the U.S. EPA weighing a large number of conflicting studies and declaring that a particular pesticide is safe to use. While that conclusion might be reasonable given the level of confidence demanded by most consumers, consumers who are particularly risk-averse might want to draw different conclusions for their own purposes given their differing standards of evidence.

One strategy for addressing these problems is to return to the principle of transparency, as discussed earlier. If scientists and policymakers could be clear enough about the values underlying their work, it would enable those with minority values to understand when they might want to pursue science that incorporates alternative judgments that more closely fit with their values (Elliott 2018). I will discuss this suggestion further in the next section.

Engagement

Engagement is a third principle that can assist in managing the value-laden judgments that arise in scientific research. Engagement consists of "efforts to interact with other people or institutions in order to exchange views, highlight problems, deliberate, and foster positive change" (Elliott 2017, 138). The scientific and political communities have recently been exploring a wide range of engagement approaches, including community-based participatory research efforts (CBPR), citizen science, citizen juries, consensus conferences, surveys, focus groups, and so on. CBPR and citizen science are particularly appropriate in environmental health contexts, where members of the public tend to be motivated and interested in pursuing research to address their concerns (Corburn 2005; Elliott and Rosenberg 2019; Lichtveld et al. 2016).

When community members are involved in research efforts, they can help guide value judgments in ways that serve their priorities. Even when they are not directly involved in research, engagement efforts with citizens can serve as powerful procedures for identifying democratic values so that scientists can take these values into account when doing research (Schroeder 2021). Finally, even if it is not clear that an engagement effort has succeeded in identifying the values that are most widely shared or democratic, it can at least help uncover important value judgments so that scientists and policymakers can be more thoughtful about how they approach those judgments.

Nevertheless, an important drawback is that the outcomes of engagement efforts depend a great deal on how they are structured. If important stakeholders are not represented, or if power imbalances are not appropriately addressed, or if the information provided to participants is framed in problematic ways, then engagement can end up being deeply problematic and misleading. Thus, while engagement efforts are important, they cannot completely replace other approaches for handling value judgments in science (Kourany 2018).

Next steps

The preceding section highlighted three principles that can help environmental health scientists to manage the value judgments associated with their work in a responsible fashion. It is clear, however, that these principles are not a panacea. They all have weaknesses, and they all deserve greater specification and elaboration. In this section, I would like to focus further attention on one of these principles—transparency—to show how environmental health scientists might move forward in the future to use it more successfully for addressing the intrinsic ethical issues associated with their research. Admittedly, because of "fixed" value judgments and one-shot science (discussed in the last section), transparency will never be sufficient by itself to solve all the ethical issues involving value judgments in science, but it is still a particularly important principle.

Transparency is important partly because even if researchers try to make value judgments in ways that are ethically and socially responsible (as the principle of representativeness recommends), and even if they elicit broad input on their value judgments (as the principle of engagement recommends), others are still bound to question the appropriateness of their judgments. Transparency allows those who disagree with the judgments to pursue alternative lines of analysis that rest on different value judgments. Therefore, transparency provides a means for addressing the deep pluralism about values that exists in contemporary societies.

Another reason for pursuing creative transparency initiatives at the present time is that they are likely to receive uptake and support because of broader trends in the scientific community. In recent years, major scientific societies and academies have been calling for science to be more open, and this resonates with the effort to make value judgments in science more transparent (see, for example, Royal Society 2012; NAS 2018). Open science can incorporate a variety of initiatives, including efforts to publish in open-access sources, to make all data underlying studies openly available, to provide access to research materials and computer code, to "register" the methodology for studies before performing them, and to make all results known whether or not they support one's hypothesis (see, for example, Nosek et al. 2015). Much of the motivation for the open science movement has come from those who want to speed scientific innovation and ensure the reproducibility of scientific results. Nevertheless, an additional goal has been to make scientific research more accessible and usable for members of the public, and this goal accords with the effort to promote transparency about value judgments (Elliott and Resnik 2019).

Given the range of different groups who make use of environmental health information, it will be important to pursue a wide range of different strategies for promoting transparency. This range of strategies is needed because, as noted in the last section, different groups of people care about different value judgments, and they need varying levels of information in order to understand the judgments that matter to them. For example, scientists who are experts in the subject under investigation can typically identify important value judgments for themselves as long as the data and the methods underlying scientific studies are made openly available to them. Transparency about data and methods is already being promoted by the open science movement. However, this kind of transparency is unlikely to be helpful for members of the public who care about a topic but who are not scientific experts (Elliott and Resnik 2019). Moreover, for their decision-making purposes it might not be important to identify all the judgments that scientific experts would care about; members of the public might care primarily about the *implications* of value judgments rather than about the judgments themselves. For example, most people are likely to be satisfied with information about whether recent studies of environmental threats are more likely to have overestimated or underestimated the risks associated with those threats.

A number of strategies can be used to help clarify value judgments and their implications for non-specialists, including policymakers and members of the public (see Elliott and Resnik 2019). First, when scientists do environmental health research that is relevant to the public, they can discuss their major results and provide context to help non-specialists interpret their results (including crucial value judgments) in accessible online venues like The Conversation (https://theconversation.com/). Universities can encourage this kind of work by rewarding it in their criteria for reappointment, promotion, and tenure. Second, scientists and scholars working in related fields (e.g., history, philosophy, and sociology of science) can collaborate to identify and communicate about important value judgments involved in research projects (e.g., Schuurbiers and Fisher 2009). Funding agencies can play an important role in encouraging these sorts of collaborations. Third, journalists can engage in "critical science journalism" designed to clarify important judgments for members of the public (see, for example, Angler 2017; Elliott 2019). Fourth, as discussed briefly in the previous section, scientists and non-specialists can collaborate in community-based participatory research projects (CBPR) and citizen science initiatives, which can highlight important judgments and give members of the public opportunities to understand and influence them (Corburn 2005; Ottinger and Cohen 2011). Fifth, government agencies can collaborate with scientists and stakeholders to design initiatives for making their data and results understandable and assessable for the purposes of non-specialists (Royal Society 2012). The U.S. National

Aeronautics and Space Administration (NASA) has engaged in several creative initiatives of this sort; one of them, the Health and Air Quality Assessment Team (HAQAST), helps stakeholders answer environmental health questions using NASA data (Holloway et al. 2018). Sixth, large nongovernmental organizations (NGOs) like the Environmental Defense Fund (EDF) or the Natural Resources Defense Council (NRDC) can use their expert scientists to analyze research results and help clarify judgments that are likely to matter to their constituents.

This list of strategies for transparency illustrates how promoting intrinsic ethics in environmental health research will require system-level thinking and efforts to incorporate multiple stakeholders. Scientists cannot achieve transparency about value judgments on their own; they need to work with scholars from other fields, as well as community members, journalists, government agencies, and NGOs. The same dynamics are obviously present when developing and implementing efforts at engagement. Even achieving representativeness will require more than just the efforts of individual scientists. To make wise choices about value judgments, scientists will often need to work in interdisciplinary teams (NRC 2015); they will need guidance from community members; they will need systems of ethical codes, guidelines, and standards to guide their work (Resnik and Elliott 2019; Kourany 2010); and they will need scientific societies and advisory bodies to keep revisiting these codes, guidelines, and standards so they remain responsive to emerging issues and concerns (Elliott 2016). Thus, promoting intrinsic ethics in environmental health research will be a complex project requiring a variety of collaborative efforts.

Conclusion

This chapter has argued for an expansive characterization of research ethics for environmental health. Using Tuana's concept of intrinsic ethics, it has shown that many of the cognitive aspects of environmental health research—including the formulation of research questions, the design of studies, the analysis and interpretation of data, and the communication of results—are ethically significant insofar as they incorporate value judgments that have consequences for society. The environmental health research community needs to develop systems for handling these judgments in a responsible fashion. The principles of transparency, representativeness, and engagement can provide guidance for developing the needed systems. However, all three principles require further specification and development. This chapter suggested concrete strategies for promoting transparency so that information about value judgments can be provided not only to expert scientists but also to non-specialists. In order to address the intrinsic ethical issues associated with environmental health research, it will be important to keep exploring these sorts of multifaceted strategies that incorporate multiple individuals and institutions in efforts to handle value judgments responsibly.

References

Angler, M.W. 2017. *Science Journalism: An Introduction*. New York: Routledge.

Betz, G. 2013. "In defence of the value-free ideal." *European Journal for Philosophy of Science* 3: 207–220.

Biddle, J. and Winsberg, E. 2010. "Value judgements and the estimation of uncertainty in climate modeling." In P.D. Magnus and J. Busch (eds.), *New Waves in Philosophy of Science*. New York: Palgrave-Macmillan, pp. 172–197.

Brown, J.R. 2010. "One-shot science." In Hans Radder (ed.), *The Commodification of Academic Research*. Pittsburgh, PA: University of Pittsburgh Press, pp. 90–109.

Brown, M. 2018. "Weaving value judgment into the tapestry of science." *Philosophy, Theory & Practice in Biology* 10: 10. http://dx.doi.org/10.3998/ptpbio. 16039257.0010.010

Brown, M. 2020. *Science and Moral Imagination: A New Ideal for Values in Science*. Pittsburgh, PA: University of Pittsburgh Press.

Corburn, J. 2005. *Street Science: Community Knowledge and Environmental Health Justice*. Cambridge: MIT Press.

Douglas, H. 2009. *Science, Policy, and the Value-Free Ideal*. Pittsburgh, PA: University of Pittsburgh Press.

Douglas, H. 2013. "The value of cognitive values." *Philosophy of Science* 80: 796–806.

Douglas, H. 2016. "Values in science." In P. Humphreys (ed.), *The Oxford Handbook of the Philosophy of Science*. New York: Oxford University Press, pp. 609–630.

Douglas, H. 2017. "Why inductive risk requires values in science." In K. Elliott and D. Steel (eds.), *Current Controversies in Values and Science*. New York: Routledge, pp. 81–93.

Elliott, K. 2008. "Scientific judgment and the limits of conflict-of-interest policies." *Accountability in Research* 15: 1–29.

Elliott, K. 2011. *Is a Little Pollution Good for You? Incorporating Societal Values in Environmental Research*. New York: Oxford University Press.

Elliott, K. 2014. "Ethical and societal values in nanotoxicology." In B. Gordijn and A.M. Cutter (eds.), *In Pursuit of Nanoethics*. Springer: Dordrecht, pp. 147–163.

Elliott, K. 2016. "Standardized study designs, value judgments, and financial conflicts of interest in research." *Perspectives on Science* 24: 529–551.

Elliott, K. 2017. *A Tapestry of Values: An Introduction to Values in Science*. New York: Oxford University Press.

Elliott, K. 2018. "A tapestry of values: Response to my critics." *Philosophy, Theory, and Practice in Biology* 10: 11.

Elliott, K. 2019. "Science journalism, value judgments, and the open science movement." *Frontiers in Communication* 4: 71.

Elliott, K. 2020. "A taxonomy of transparency in science." *Canadian Journal of Philosophy*. https://doi.org/10.1017/can.2020.21

Elliott, K. and Resnik, D. 2019. "Making open science work for science and society." *Environmental Health Perspectives* 127: 075002.

Elliott, K. and Richards, T., eds. 2017. *Exploring Inductive Risk: Case Studies of Values in Science*. New York: Oxford University Press.

Elliott, K. and Rosenber, J. 2019. "Philosophical foundations for citizen science." *Citizen Science: Theory and Practice* 4: 9.

Elliott, K. and Steel, D., eds. 2017. *Contemporary Controversies in Values and Science*. New York: Routledge.

Fernández Pinto, M. and Hicks, D.J. 2019. "Legitimizing values in regulatory science." *Environmental Health Perspectives* 127: 035001.

Havstad, J.C. and Brown, M.J. 2017. "Inductive risk, deferred decisions, and climate science advising." In K. Elliott and T. Richards (eds.), *Exploring Inductive Risk: Case Studies of Values in Science.* New York: Oxford University Press, pp. 101–125.

Holloway, T., Jacob, D.J., and Miller, D. 2018. "Short history of NASA applied science teams for air quality and health." *Journal of Applied Remote Sensing* 12: 1.

Hudson, R. 2016. "Why we should not reject the value-free ideal of science." *Perspectives on Science* 24: 167–191.

Intemann, I. 2015. "Distinguishing between legitimate and illegitimate values in climate modeling." *European Journal for Philosophy of Science* 5: 217–232.

John, S. 2015. "Inductive risk and the contexts of communication." *Synthese* 192: 79–96.

Kourany, J. 2010. *Philosophy of Science after Feminism.* New York: Oxford University Press.

Kourany, J. 2018. "Adding to the tapestry." *Philosophy, Theory, and Practice in Biology* 10: 9.

Lichtveld, M., Goldstein, B., Grattan, L., and Mundorf, C. 2016. "Then and now: Lessons learned from community-academic partnerships in environmental health research." *Environmental Health* 15: 117.

Longino, H. 1990. *Science as Social Knowledge: Values and Objectivity in Scientific Inquiry.* Princeton, NJ: Princeton University Press.

NAS (National Academies of Sciences, Engineering, and Medicine). 2018. *Open Science by Design: Realizing a Vision for 21st Century Research.* Washington, DC: National Academies Press.

NRC (National Research Council). 2015. *Enhancing the Effectiveness of Team Science.* Washington, DC: National Academies Press.

Nosek, B.A., Alter, G., Banks, G.C., Borsboom, D., Bowman, S.D., Breckler, S.J., Buck, S., Chambers, C.D., Chin, G., Christensen, G., and Contestabile, M. 2015. "Promoting an open research culture." *Science* 348: 1422–1425.

Ottinger, G. and B. Cohen, eds. 2011. *Technoscience and Environmental Justice: Expert Cultures in a Grassroots Movement.* Cambridge: MIT Press.

Resnik, D.B. and Elliott, K.C. 2019. "Value-entanglement and the integrity of scientific research." *Studies in History and Philosophy of Science.* https://doi.org/10.1016/j.shpsa.2018.12.011

Royal Society. 2012. *Science as an Open Enterprise.* London: The Royal Society.

Schroeder, S.A. 2019. "Which values should be built into economic measures?" *Economics & Philosophy* 35: 521–536.

Schroeder, S.A. 2020. "Values in science: Ethical vs. political approaches." *Canadian Journal of Philosophy.* https://doi.org/10.1017/can.2020.41

Schroeder, S.A. 2021. "Democratic values: A better foundation for public trust in science." *British Journal for Philosophy of Science.* https://doi.org/10.1093/bjps/axz023

Schuurbiers, D. and Fisher, E. 2009. "Lab-scale intervention." *EMBO Reports* 10: 424–427.

Shamoo, A.E. and Resnik, D.B. 2015. *Responsible Conduct of Research*, 3rd ed. New York: Oxford University Press.

Shrader-Frechette, K.S. 1994. *Ethics of Scientific Research.* Lanham, MD: Rowman and Littlefield.

Steel, D. 2010. "Epistemic values and the argument from inductive risk." *Philosophy of Science* 77: 14–34.

Tuana, N. 2010. "Leading with ethics, aiming for policy: New opportunities for philosophy of science." *Synthese* 177: 471–492.

Vandenberg, L.N., Hunt, P.A. and Gore, A.C. 2019. "Endocrine disruptors and the future of toxicology testing—Lessons from CLARITY–BPA." *Nature Reviews Endocrinology.*

Ward, Z. 2021. "On value-laden science." *Studies in History and Philosophy of Science* 85: 54–62.

Wilholt, T. 2013. "Epistemic trust in science." *The British Journal for the Philosophy of Science* 64: 233–253.

11 The flow of values in environmental risk assessments

Per Wikman-Svahn

Scientific assessments play an important role in managing environmental risks in society, and choices made by scientists and experts involved in making these assessments can have surprisingly critical policy implications. Here, this phenomenon, which I call "value-inertia," is conceptualized and discussed. Value-inertia is of high relevance for environmental health, for example, when assessing the health impacts of environmental releases of toxic substances and how to make decisions based on such information.

The chapter is structured as follows. First, I introduce a model of the steps from science to policy. In the following section, I expound the concept of value-inertia using examples of assessments of climate change and sea-level rise. Then, I discuss the objection that value-inertia need not be any problem, because scientific values ought to influence policy. Finally, I discuss how different actors in science and policy can address issues of value-inertia.

A model of the information flow from science to policy

Hansson and Aven (2014) discuss the philosophical basis of risk analysis as a scientific activity and introduce a simple model of "the information flow in the process in which science is used as a base for decision-making" (p. 1177). Hansson and Aven's (2014) model is graphically represented in Figure 11.1 and will henceforth be called the Model, in short.

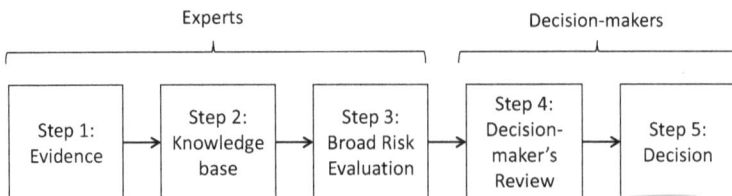

Figure 11.1 A model of the flow of information from science to decision-making. The arrows represent the flow of information between the different steps. Adapted from Hansson and Aven (2014).

DOI: 10.4324/9780429318436-16

The information flow from science to a decision in the Model starts with *Step 1: Evidence*, where scientific information is produced by experts and published and made available for other experts and the general public (e.g., publications in peer-reviewed scientific journals). The evidence is used in *Step 2: Knowledge-base*, which is "the collection of all 'truths' (legitimate truth claims) and beliefs that the majority of scientists in the area take as given in further research in the field" (Hansson & Aven 2014, p. 1177). In *Step 3: Broad risk evaluation*, "the knowledge base is evaluated, and summary judgment is reached on the risks and uncertainties involved in the case under investigation" (p. 1177). While Step 3 is typically done by independent experts, often an additional assessment is made before deciding. Hence, *Step 4: Decision-makers review*, where decision-makers "combine the risk information they have received with information from other sources and on other topics" (p. 1178). Thus, in Step 4 broader considerations of the decision-maker, not covered in the previous step, are added to the evaluation before the final step—*Step 5: Decision*.[1]

The focus of Hansson and Aven (2014) is on Step 3, for which they say that the experts working in this step have "to take the values of the decision-makers into account" (p. 1177) because the evaluation often is so "entwined with scientific issues" that it becomes impossible for the experts to defer the value judgments to decision-makers.

However, it is not clear exactly how experts should take the values of the decision-makers into account. Hansson and Aven (2014) do not discuss it in detail, other than stating that experts need to make a careful distinction between the "scientific burden of proof" and the "practical burden of proof" for the decision (p. 1177). They also note that "the value component of risk decisions should be displayed as clearly as possible" (2014, p. 1181). Similar requirements of transparency are standard whenever the role of values in science is discussed (see, for example, Elliott 2017). However, transparency can be tough to achieve in practice, which is precisely the reason why experts should take the values of the decision-makers into account.

But even if experts can take the values of the decision-makers into account when producing their assessments, the result might still be influenced by value judgments made in the previous steps (Steps 1 and 2 in the Model). In the next section, this phenomenon is conceptualized and discussed.

Value-inertia in the steps from science to decision

Value-inertia is the phenomenon that some choices, and therefore the values influencing these choices, made at earlier steps in the process from science to policy, tend to have critical impacts in later stages. I suggest that this phenomenon is widespread and that it deserves to be conceptualized and counteracted. In essence, value-inertia is the tendency that the influence of values has lasting effects (see Figure 11.2).

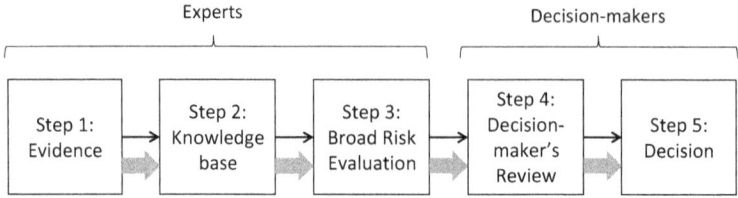

Figure 11.2 Value-inertia in the process from science to decision. The fat arrows illustrate the influence of value judgments.

Below I provide case studies of how choices at previous stages in the process from science to decision can have critical effects at later stages. The values that guided these choices, therefore, had lasting consequences "down-stream" in the process of information flow from science to a decision. Value-inertia seems important to highlight both for the theory of values in science and policy and for practical policy purposes in risk assessments.

In what follows, I will discuss value-inertia using examples from assessments of future climate change and sea-level rise.

Step 1: evidence

In Step 1, scientific knowledge is produced and made available for other researchers and the public (e.g., in scientific publications). Already at this step, choices are made that can have far-reaching consequences. Here I will exemplify this with critical choices in scientific assessments of future climate change.

A fundamental problem when assessing future climate change is that we don't know how much greenhouse gases there will be in the atmosphere in the future, as this is contingent on a large number of uncertain social factors.[2] These social factors are highly uncertain on a timescale of several decades, which makes it in practice impossible to "predict" future climate change on these timescales.

In climate change science, the standard practice to deal with the uncertainty in future concentrations of greenhouse gases is not to make "predictions," but instead to make "projections," which are contingent on future "scenarios" or "pathways" of emissions of greenhouse gases in the atmosphere. Scientists can, therefore, avoid making choices on uncertain assumptions, such as the social factors discussed above. However, climate scientists still need to select which scenarios to use to base their calculations and model results on, especially what range of emission scenarios to use.

In recent years, most studies on future climate change impacts make projections contingent on scenarios called "Representative Concentration Pathways," or "RCPs" (Van Vuuren et al. 2011). There are four main RCPs:

RCP2.6, RCP4.5, RCP6, and RCP8.5.[3] The choice of this set of scenarios to use as a basis for making climate projections, in particular, the highest and the lowest in the range of the RCP scenarios, is highly consequential, as we will see below.

But who is making these choices, and why? The scientists making a climate study, could, in theory, choose any particular emission scenario as an input to their climate model. However, in practice, the choice of what emission scenarios to use is circumscribed. In recent years, the option to use the RCP scenarios is almost taken as given in climate science, and any other choice would need justification when writing up the study for publication in a scientific journal. Moreover, there is scientific value in that many studies use the same scenarios, which enables comparability between different studies.[4]

I am not criticizing the choice to use the RCPs. On the contrary, I think it is entirely appropriate to handle the fundamental uncertainty in future global emissions of greenhouse gases using different assumptions. However, the point I want to make is that the choice to use the range of these four particular emission scenarios is a critical choice, which has consequences down the line.

Step 2: knowledge base

The second step in the Model is the "knowledge base." An excellent example of this is the general Assessment Reports produced by the Intergovernmental Panel on Climate Change (IPCC). The IPCC's Assessment Reports are developed by a large group of international experts, volunteering their time and efforts to produce comprehensive reports of the knowledge base regarding climate change. Similar assessments are made in other areas of relevance for environmental health. For example, in assessments of the effects of ionizing radiation, there are reports on the knowledge base from influential organizations such as the International Commission on Radiological Protection (ICRP) and the United Nations Scientific Committee on the Effects of Atomic Radiation (UNSCEAR). Here I will use the example of future sea-level rise and discuss critical choices made by the IPCC when assessing and communicating sea-level science.

One critical choice by the IPCC is the use of the RCP scenarios to present the results in the report. The assessment report from the IPCC from 2013 projected that global mean sea levels at the end of the 21st century would likely be 0.26–0.55 m for RCP2.6 and 0.45–0.82 m for RCP8.5 (Church et al. 2013, p. 1140).[5] Note the vast difference the choice of RCP makes: the projections for the sea-level rise at the end of the century being almost twice as high for RCP8.5 compared to RCP2.6.[6]

Another critical choice by the IPCC is how it communicates the uncertainties. The IPCC uses a standardized language for communicating uncertainties (described in Mastrandrea et al. 2010). For example, the projection of sea-level rise in the 2013 report by the IPCC assuming RCP8.5 is "likely"

0.52–0.98 m by 2100 (compared to the reference period 1986–2005; Church et al. 2013, p. 1140). The use of the term "likely" means that the authors of the IPCC report estimate that the probability of the actual number falling outside this range is higher than 66%.

My point is that the choice of the "likely" uncertainty interval by the IPCC authors is a choice, which has implications for how people are interpreting the report, as will be discussed in connection to the next step.

For assessments of future sea-level rise by 2100, the choice of an uncertainty interval has an even more significant effect than the emission scenarios. For an example of this, we can look at another comprehensive climate assessment: the 2017 U.S. national climate assessment (Sweet et al. 2017). Interestingly the U.S. report provides a greater uncertainty range. The "intermediate scenario" in the U.S. report assuming RCP8.5 is 1.0 m by 2100 (compared to the reference year 2000), with an assessed probability of 17% exceeding this level (Sweet et al. 2017, Tables 12.1 and 12.4), which is comparable to the IPCC's "likely" projection for RCP8.5 of 0.98 m by 2100.[7] However, the U.S. report also provides more extreme scenarios of sea-level rise by 2100: 1.5 m, 2.0 m, and 2.5 m, with respective probabilities of exceeding these levels of 1.3%, 0.3%, and 0.1%. Thus, the U.S. report goes far beyond the uncertainty range of the IPCC report.

What were the values influencing the choices made by the authors of the IPCC report and the U.S. report? The choice by the IPCC authors to state their findings on future sea-level rise in the "likely" interval instead of a greater uncertainty interval (the IPCC language of "very likely" would, for example, imply a greater than 90% probability) can perhaps be explained in the context of the IPCC's objectives, for example, consistency with how other climate impacts are communicated in other parts of the report. But what is important to note is that the effect of these choices results in different ways to communicate the knowledge base regarding future sea-level rise. This has consequences in the next step in the process, from science to decision-making, as I will describe below.

Step 3: broad risk evaluation

Assessments from the knowledge base can rarely be used directly in decision-making. In the case of future flooding, the answers to the question of how much future sea levels will rise at a particular geographic location are not the focus of the IPCC reports. In most countries, these local and regional assessments are produced by national weather and climate agencies. The task to provide local flooding risk assessments and how these might be impacted by climate change and sea-level rise can be seen as Step 3 in the Model. However, the expert assessments in Step 3 depend on the results from the previous steps and, thus, are subject to the consequences of past choices and the values influencing these choices—what I call value-inertia.

A case study of this is the assessment of coastal flooding made for the Swedish Civil Contingencies Agency (MSB) as a basis for identifying areas with a high risk of flooding in Sweden (MSB 2018). The assessment was made for the decision-makers at MSB by experts from the Swedish Meteorological and Hydrological Institute (SMHI). The evaluation was based on two sea-level scenarios for Sweden in the year 2100, one assuming RCP4.5 and one RCP8.5 scenario. Here we again see how the choice of emission scenarios (from Steps 1 and 2) have lasting effects. Moreover, the extreme scenario in the Swedish assessment is based on the IPCC projections of global mean sea level, using the highest reported "likely" level in the IPCC report: 0.98 m by 2100 assuming RCP8.5 (Nerheim et al. 2017).

This case illustrates how previous choices by the IPCC to provide projections based on the RCP8.5 scenario and the "likely" uncertainty range had direct consequences for the Swedish assessment of areas with substantial flooding risk. It seems plausible that if the IPCC had used some other scenario for the highest projections instead of RCP8.5 (e.g., hypothetical emission scenarios called "RCP7.5" or "RCP9.0"), or if the IPCC had chosen to provide projections based on something else than the "likely" interval (e.g., the "very likely" interval), then the Swedish scenarios would have been different. Similar dependencies on the IPCC assessments are probably common in many other countries all over the world.

Steps 4 and 5: the decision-maker's review and the final decision

Decisions in policy are rarely made purely based on the results from the assessment in Step 3, as other issues typically have to be considered in a decision. It is not uncommon that the decision-maker also employs 'own' experts in the field. Decision-makers might even choose to get a "second opinion" by commissioning another study. In Step 4, the decision-makers thus have an opportunity to mitigate some of the problems of value-inertia. For example, they might choose to assign additional margins to the assessments or add a "safety factor." This is often the case if the decision-makers are aware that there are problems in previous studies or uncertainties that are not accurately managed in these studies. But even without such suspicion, decision-makers might find it prudent to add some extra margin of safety. An example of this is the recommendations on the lowest level of the ground for new buildings due to flooding risks in the Stockholm region in Sweden that adds a "safety factor" (Carlsson-Kanyama et al. 2019).

However, even if a safety factor is used in the decision-makers' review, that safety-factor is set in relation to the previous assessment. Moreover, also if the decision-makers' review could, in theory, revise the assessments based on an understanding of critical value judgments, this is not always done. Improving the quality of the decision-makers' reviews to better consider the values of the decision-makers and stakeholders is vital to improving environmental risk assessment and management. Some suggestions on how this can be done are discussed in the final section of this chapter.

Why value–inertia can be a problem

Someone might object and say that it doesn't seem to be any problem that scientific values influence decision-making. The objection is that this is something that we should strive for; policy ought to be based on science, and therefore only "scientific values" ought to influence assessments of environmental risks.

I agree that decision-making should be based on science. However, the problem arises when some value judgments in science have a critical impact on policy decisions in inappropriate ways. Value–inertia might not always be a problem, but it can be for some reasons. One reason is that arbitrary value judgments might influence policy decisions. Previous choices and values are, of course, not random in the context in which they originate. However, from a particular decision-makers' perspective, say a municipality considering what land to develop or not, choices and the values made "up-stream" by the scientists and experts of the IPCC (e.g., what RCP scenario to use or what uncertainty interval to communicate) are in practice almost arbitrary.

Another reason why value–inertia is problematic has to do with responsibility and accountability. If decisions are significantly impacted by choices made by experts in previous steps and the values influencing these choices, then it becomes unclear who bears the responsibility for the decisions. The solution to counteract this problem is to moderate the expert assessment (in Step 3 or 4), by the influence of values from the decision-context (see Figure 11.3).

However, this introduces another problem: How can we make sure that the influence of values on the expert assessment is justified and does not involve inappropriate modification of the science? The question is, how should values be allowed to influence the expert assessment? This is a difficult question, which does not have a simple answer. Hansson and Aven (2014) note that experts working in Step 3 "regularly operate in a 'no man's land' between science and policy, and it is no surprise that they often find themselves criticized on value-based grounds" (p. 1177).

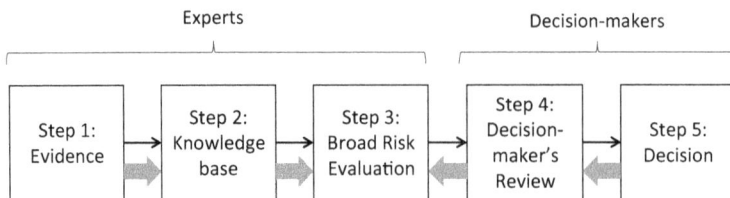

Figure 11.3 Influence of values from the decision-makers to the risk assessment.

The experts working in Step 3 or 4 must respect and not distort the science and the facts. Still, they must, at the same time, be independent and know how values of the decision context may legitimately moderate the assessment. Exactly how this can and ought to be done is an important question, which has to be discussed elsewhere. Many of the insights and lessons for the discourse on values in science likely apply to expert assessments (in Steps 3 and 4). Still, particular circumstances need to be considered for experts in their role as experts informing decision-makers and policy (see Chapter 10; also Vareman & Persson 2010; Steele 2012; Gundersen 2018).

What can be done to reduce the problems of value-inertia?

Decision-makers need to be aware of value-inertia and that the assessments may be affected by the phenomenon. Decision-makers should, therefore, try to identify critical value judgments from previous steps. This can, of course, be difficult, which makes the "decision-makers' review" (Step 4) even more critical. Ideally, the decision-makers' review should highlight vital value judgments and their implications on the assessments. However, overruling high-profile and authoritative international and national assessments may be difficult and contentious. Still, the alternative of just taking these assessments as they are, off the shelf so to speak, opens the gate for value-inertia to have a direct influence on policy decisions.

Not all organizations can afford to have their experts in house or to commission new assessments. Here larger organizations, such as professional societies and national governmental agencies, have essential roles to play, for example, to commission studies that are of high scientific quality but at the same time consider a wide range of different stakeholders' and decision-makers' interests. National governmental authorities with responsibility in one area could influence other federal regulatory authorities in other areas to make studies that take their interests and values into account. More interaction and collaboration between different stakeholders, therefore, seem beneficial to help reduce the problems of value-inertia.

Experts producing reports that are used as a basis for policy (in Step 3 in the Model) could also benefit from being aware of value-inertia. Experts should know that some value judgments make more sense in some contexts than in others. The experts, therefore, need to make their value judgments that are adapted to the needs of the decision-makers and stakeholders. But how should the experts do this?

A commonly stated requirement is that value judgments should be made transparent for the decision-makers. However, this is easier said than done in most cases. The problem is that a large number of choices need to be made in an expert assessment. For example, what studies to include or exclude, how to weigh different studies, how to communicate the findings, and so on. In practice, it is difficult and unpractical to document all these choices and the reasons for making these choices.

Because experts cannot be completely transparent about every value judgment that goes into their assessment, experts have an even greater responsibility for making the "right choices." However, making the right decisions can be difficult, especially as there is no consensus on how values ought to influence expert assessments. One way to deal with this challenge is to create forums in which the experts can discuss these issues openly among peers. Conferences of professional organizations can play a significant role in enabling such discussions.

Another way to make it easier to make the right value judgments is when the experts have a good understanding of the needs and values of the decision-makers and the stakeholders involved. In general, more iterative processes seem preferable. An iterative process enables the co-production of knowledge so that the assessment can be based on the values and interests of the decision-makers and stakeholders. Of course, this might not always be possible or practicable and will likely take more time and be more expensive. In the end, a higher cost and trouble in the expert assessment must be weighed against the risks and costs of making bad policy decisions, based on evaluations that are poorly adapted to the values of the decision-makers and the stakeholders.

Finally, what can scientists and experts producing scientific evidence (Step 1) or producing comprehensive reviews and syntheses of state of the art in different scientific topics (Step 2) do in light of value-inertia?

A good start would be to aim for greater transparency. But, as I have argued above, transparency is not enough, because choices to exclude issues in a study or how to report the results can also be seen as value judgments subject to value-inertia. So even better than transparency would be to consider a wide range of possible stakeholder interests and values.

For example, if scientists have reason to believe that some stakeholders are interested in the extreme outcomes of a study, then scientists could choose to vary parameters and assumptions that have a significant impact on the extremes. Scientists could then also decide to present their results over larger uncertainty ranges. The potential for value-inertia creates responsibilities for scientists and experts to consider the consequences of their choices and how to make the implications of these choices more clear for others, both experts and non-experts.

Some might see this as opposed to the view that science ought to be free from social values, the so-called "value-free ideal" of science (see e.g., Betz 2013, Douglas 2016). However, taking values into account does not necessarily imply that we allow wishful thinking to influence scientific results.

Taking values in science seriously, being transparent about these values, and representing different sets of values, will lead to both more usable and better science. I have argued that value-inertia is an important phenomenon and suggested ways of how the potential problems of value-inertia can be reduced. Most importantly, we need a better understanding of value-inertia and the flow of values from science to policy.

Notes

1 Hansson and Aven acknowledge that the model involves simplification and that there are other flows of information, for instance, questions from decision-makers to experts and feedback from risk assessors to scientists.
2 Including factors such as global population; land use; and which technologies will be used in energy production, transportation, industry, and agriculture, which in turn depends on technological, economic, political, and social developments, and so on.
3 The numbers in the names of the scenarios represent the warming effects of greenhouse gases in the atmosphere captured in a measure called "radiative forcing" (measured in Watts per square meter). For example, the RCP with the lowest concentrations of greenhouse gases in year 2100 is RCP2.6, which describes a future with rapidly decreasing greenhouse emissions (after a peak early in the century) and resulting in an aggregate radiative forcing of 2.6 W/m^2 by year 2100. On the other end of the range, RCP8.5 describes a future with rapidly rising emissions of greenhouse gases throughout the end of the century resulting in a radiative forcing by year 2100 of 8.5 W/m^2.
4 This is especially important when comparing different climate models used by different research groups. For climate science, the very influential "Coupled Model Intercomparison Project (CMIP)" (Eyring et al. 2016) provides guidelines of input and output for climate models and is used as a basis for international assessments, including the Intergovernmental Panel on Climate Change (IPCC) reports.
5 The numbers are for the period 2081–2100, compared to the reference period 1986–2005.
6 The IPCC also influenced the production of the RCP scenarios from the start (van Vuuren et al. 2011), thus creating a "value-influence" in the other direction.
7 If we assume a symmetric probability distribution for the "likely" range used by the IPCC.

References

Betz, G. (2013). In defence of the value free ideal. *European Journal for Philosophy of Science*, *3*(2), 207–220.

Carlsson-Kanyama, A., Wikman-Svahn, P., & Mossberg Sonnek, K. (2019).: "We want to know where the line is": Comparing current planning for future sea-level rise with three core principles of robust decision support approaches., *Journal of Environmental Planning and Management*,. *62*(8), 1339–1358.

Church, J. A. et al. (2013). Sea level change. In *Climate Change 2013: The Physical Science Basis*, T.F. Stocker et al. (Eds.). Cambridge and New York: Cambridge University Press. 1137–1216.

Douglas, H. (2016). Values in science. In *The Oxford Handbook of Philosophy of Science*, P. Humphrey (Ed.). 609–632. New York: Oxford University Press.

Elliott, K. C. (2017). *A Tapestry of Values: An Introduction to Values in Science*. New York: Oxford University Press.

Eyring, V., Bony, S., Meehl, G. A., Senior, C. A., Stevens, B., Stouffer, R. J., & Taylor, K. E. (2016). Overview of the Coupled Model Intercomparison Project Phase 6 (CMIP6) experimental design and organization. *Geoscientific Model Development (Online)*, *9*(LLNL-JRNL-736881).

Gundersen, T. (2018). Scientists as experts: A distinct role? *Studies in History and Philosophy of Science Part A*, *69*, 52–59.

Hansson, S. O., & Aven, T. (2014). Is risk analysis scientific? *Risk Analysis, 34*(7), 1173–1183.

Mastrandrea, M. D., Field, C. B., Stocker, T. F., Edenhofer, O., Ebi, K., Frame, D. J., Held, H., Kriegler, E., Mach, K. J., Matschoss, P. R., Plattner, G.-K., Yohe, G. W., & Zwiers, F. W. (2010). *Guidance Note for Lead Authors of the IPCC Fifth Assessment Report on Consistent Treatment of Uncertainties.* Intergovernmental Panel on Climate Change (IPCC). Available at <http://www.ipcc.ch>.

MSB (2018). Översyn av områden med betydande översvämningsrisk. Publikationsnummer MSB1152-Januari 2018.

Nerheim, S., Schöld, S., Persson, G., & Sjöström, Å. (2017). Framtida havsnivåer i Sverige. SMHI Klimatologi Nr 48.

Steele, K. (2012). The scientist qua policy advisor makes value judgments. *Philosophy of Science, 79*(5), 893–904.

Sweet, W. V. et al. (2017). Sea level rise. In *Climate Science Special Report: Fourth National Climate Assessment, Volume I*, Wuebbles, D. J. et al. (Eds.). Washington, DC: U.S. Global Change Research Program. 333–363.

Van Vuuren, D. P., Edmonds, J., Kainuma, M., Riahi, K., Thomson, A., Hibbard, K., Hurtt, G. C., Kram, T., Krey, V., Lamarque, J. F., & Masui, T. (2011). The representative concentration pathways: An overview. *Climatic Change, 109*(1–2), 5.

Vareman, N., & Persson, J. (2010). Why separate risk assessors and risk managers? Further external values affecting the risk assessor qua risk assessor. *Journal of Risk Research, 13*(5), 687–700.

12 Principles of research ethics for environmental health – historical development and current trends

Friedo Zölzer

Environmental health as well as research ethics have been around for quite some time, but the specifics of ethics for environmental health research have not been given much attention until about 20 years ago. In 2003, the journal *Environmental Health Perspectives* published a 'mini-monograph' on 'Ethics in Environmental Health', which the editor claimed to be 'largely unchartered territory' (Parascandola, 2003). The six papers making up the monograph addressed questions that were to 'attract the attention of regulators, politicians, private industry, and the general public', but they also drew attention to specific ethical challenges with which environmental health researchers would be confronted. In addition to these papers and a few others published independently around the same time, another valuable resource is Chapter 11 in Resnik's standard work of 2012 on *Environmental Health Ethics*, which discussed 'Environmental Health Research Involving Human Subjects' and mentions further relevant publications. Again, although some of the papers cited were from before 2003, none expressly named environmental health research ethics as their topic. Finally, some relevant material can be found in two compilations of papers presented respectively at the 2nd and 3rd International Symposium on Ethics of Environmental Health in Budweis, Czech Republic, and published under the titles of 'Ethics of Environmental Health' (Zölzer and Meskens, 2017) and 'Environmental Health Risks – Ethical Aspects' (Zölzer and Meskens, 2019).

What follows here is an overview of the historical development and current trends in the area, with particular emphasis on the principles which have been suggested in the course of time as guidance for ethically sound research on environmental health. It will become obvious that these principles are very much the same as for the practice of environmental health (or for public health in general), although there is a certain diversity of views when it comes to their application in research. Both the 'specification' of the general principles to the field of environmental health and the 'balancing' between them when they seem to be in conflict require discussion. It is more and more understood that this is something which cannot be done by environmental health researchers alone but that it needs to involve all stakeholders and would also profit from a greater awareness of cross-cultural commonalities and differences.

DOI: 10.4324/9780429318436-17

Some early history

When searching for the historical origins of environmental health, one is usually referred to a number of authors of the 19th century, who will be discussed shortly. Long before that, however, there was obviously some understanding of the relationship between human health and environmental factors. In antiquity, Hippocrates (460–370 BC) and Pliny the Elder (24–79) described work-related heavy-metal poisoning (Abrams, 2001). One of the most prominent figures of medieval medicine, Avicenna (aka Ibn Sina; 980–1037), included air, water, location, housing, and occupation among the factors that affect the physical condition of humans (Al Khayat, 1997). Significant knowledge about the effects of environmental factors on human health was gained during the early modern period through the study of occupational diseases. Ulrich Ellenbog wrote about the health effects of working with coal and heavy metals in 1473 (Koelsch and Zoepfl, 1927); Agricola (Georg Bauer) in 1556 (Schiffer, 1977) and Paracelsus (Theophrastus Bombastus von Hohenheim) in 1567 (Müller, 2013) described the occurrence of chronic lung diseases among miners; Bernardino Ramazzini in 1700 (Cave, 1940) talked of a whole series of occupational diseases and their causes (which is why he is often called the 'father of occupational medicine'); and Percival Pott in 1775 (Pott, 1775) discussed the role of soot in the development of scrotal cancer in chimney sweeps. Much of this was presumably based on anecdotal observations rather than systematic research, and nothing can be stated with certainty about the ethical principles by which these early occupational health scientists may have been guided.

Scientific investigation on the influence of certain factors in our living and working environment, that is, epidemiology in the modern sense, indeed began in the first half of the 19th century. Charles Turner Thackrah (1795–1833) explored the connection between workplace conditions and certain diseases (Thackrah, 1832). A little later, Edwin Chadwick (1800–1890) undertook research that focused primarily on the health effects of housing conditions (Chadwick, 1843). Both had significant influence on British legislation. The most prominent pioneer of occupational health and safety legislation in the United States was Alice Hamilton (1869–1970), who conducted ground-breaking research on a range of toxic substances in the workplace and the diseases they caused (Hamilton, 1943). In Germany and Austria, the leading specialists on occupational health were Ludwig Hirt (1844–1910) and Ludwig Teleky (1872–1957), who both conducted research into the health effects of working conditions and fought for the implementation of more worker-friendly legislations (Müller and Milles, 1984).

Even at that stage of what is now called 'Environmental and occupational health', there is no evidence for any detailed consideration and discussion of research ethics. What can be said is that the English and German pioneers in the field seem to have been motivated by high ideals, in particular by the wish to alleviate the hardships of the working class, the poor and needy, and the underprivileged. Thackrah, in a talk which he gave at the Leeds Philosophical and Literary Society as a young man, mentions our 'moral responsibility' not to sit idle but to 'exert ourselves … for the advancement of human knowledge and human happiness' (Thackrah, 1821). Of Chadwick, it is known that he was a close friend and follower of Jeremy Bentham, the founder of utilitarianism, and that he saw his endeavours as a means to contribute to the 'Greatest happiness for the greatest number of people' (Ringen, 1979). Hamilton came from a progressive and socially engaged family and was guided by her sense of responsibility for the less well-to-do, with a deep appreciation of the connection between health and social issues (Forrest Weber, 1995). For Hirt, a particularly worrying fact was that workers were not sufficiently informed about occupational health risks, and he therefore shared the results of his studies in a language accessible to all (Schiebelsberger, 2009). Teleky emphasised that the physician's care for the needy should not be oriented primarily towards ensuring their operational capability but rather towards establishing social justice (Hien, 2011).

Admittedly, all of this cannot count as research ethics, whose beginnings must rather be traced back to clinical medicine (Rice, 2008). In the 19th century, questions about research on human subjects did raise concerns for a number of people, who recognised that a certain standard or code of conduct – one would now say ethical framework – was necessary for such activities. The German psychiatrist Albert Moll, for instance, collected 600 cases in which nontherapeutic research had been carried out on human subjects with serious ethical shortcomings, such as the lack of informed consent (Maehle, 2012). A particular infamous case was that of the German venereologist Albert Neisser, who had injected a number of women with serum from syphilis patients in a (futile) attempt to immunise them against the disease. The (Prussian) Royal Disciplinary Court for Civil Servants convicted him on the charge of not obtaining the women's consent. A public debate ensued, leading to a Prussian state directive for hospitals and clinics in 1900, which advised that nontherapeutic research could not be carried out on minors and incompetent persons, and otherwise only if 'unambiguous consent' had been given 'after proper explanation of the possible negative consequences'. The directive was not legally binding, however, and it is questionable what impact it really had. It was only in 1931, after another round of public debate, that the German government issued detailed 'guidelines for new therapy and human experimentation', which again included many 'modern' concepts such as the necessity of informed consent (Vollmann and Winau, 1996). Sadly, of course, these guidelines did not prevent doctors under the Nazi regime, which came to power two years later, from conducting horrific experiments on human subjects, especially on Jewish as well as Sinti and Roma inmates of concentration camps. Nevertheless, the fact that there was ethics of research on human subjects before the Nazi period shows that the tendency of many reviews to portray the Nuremberg trials of 1946 as the very beginning of such ethics is an overstatement.

The basis of the current framework of human-subject-related research

Of course, the Nuremberg Code was a major step forward, containing ethical standards to which physicians should have conformed and must conform when carrying out experimentation on human subjects (Moreno et al., 2017). In particular, it stipulated that

– 'the voluntary consent of the human subject is absolutely essential'; 'that the person involved should have … sufficient knowledge and comprehension … as to enable him to make an understanding and enlightened decision'; and that 'the human subject should be at liberty to bring the experiment to an end.'
– 'the experiment should be such as to yield fruitful results for the good of society, unprocurable by other methods or means of study'; that 'the experiment should be so conducted as to avoid all unnecessary physical and mental suffering and injury'; and that 'the degree of risk to be taken should never exceed that determined by the humanitarian importance of the problem to be solved by the experiment.'

In the early 1960s, efforts were made by the World Medical Association to draw up standards 'to guide physicians all over the world' on how to conduct clinical research. A draft was published in 1962, and the final document was accepted in 1964. This 'Declaration of Helsinki' does not explicitly refer to the Nuremberg Code, but is clearly based on it. There are only few differences, the most significant being that whereas the Code spoke of an 'absolute requirement' for informed consent, the new Declaration allowed consent to be given by the 'legal guardian' in cases of 'legal incapacity' (Fluss, 1999). The Declaration of Helsinki has been revised seven times, latest in 2013, and important features have been added to it, such as distributive justice and protection of the vulnerable (Malik and Foster, 2016). These are aspects of particular importance for environmental health research to be discussed in some more detail below.

The Nuremberg Code received little attention among medical researchers, up until around the time that the Declaration of Helsinki came into being. Perhaps physicians, especially in the United States, felt it was relevant only for barbarians like the Nazis, not for civilised people like themselves. In 1965, however, Henry Beecher presented a paper at a science journalist conference and a year later published a revised version of it in a leading medical journal (Beecher, 1966), where he described 22 recent cases of inappropriate medical experimentation in the United States. One case that was mentioned in his review but did not become very prominent until extensive media coverage in 1972 was the Tuskegee Syphilis Study (Baker et al., 2005). It involved withholding effective treatment for syphilis from several hundred African American men, in order to monitor the progress of the disease and thereby to gain further insight into its pathogenesis. The study subjects were not informed about their condition and were even actively misled with regard to the 'health care' they were receiving, allowing them to progress onto the tertiary stage of syphilis when it could have been prevented by known treatments at the time. Although there were a number of similar studies which turned out to have ignored the standards of medical research that should have been common by the time (Rice, 2008), this one in particular triggered a public debate in the United States which finally led to the passing of the National Research Act in 1974, U.S. Congress's first legislation regarding research on human subjects (Resnik, 2012).

One provision of the National Research Act was the creation of a 'National Commission for the Protection of Human Subjects of Biomedical and Behavioral Research' which was to develop guidelines for research on human subjects and to oversee and regulate it as well. Only four years later, the Commission issued the 'Belmont Report: Ethical Principles and Guidelines for the Protection of Human Subjects of Research' (Adashi et al., 2018). There is no need to go into details here, because this report is discussed at length in Chapter 9 of the present volume. Suffice it to say that the three principles which it stipulates very much echo the Nuremberg Code and the Declaration of Helsinki:

- Respect for persons (calling for informed consent, and protection of the vulnerable)
- Beneficence (including avoidance of harm and minimisation of risk)
- Justice (demanding a fair distribution of burdens and benefits)

Again, it has to be emphasised that what has been discussed so far refers to ethics of research involving human subjects, which is certainly relevant for ethics of environmental health research, but of course does not completely cover it. Just as medical ethics is focusing on concrete clinical situations and does not necessarily give answers to questions coming up in the context of public health, research ethics for environmental health requires a shift of attention away from individual human subjects to whole populations (Soskolne and Sieswerda, 1998; Childress et al., 2002).

Ethical principles for environmental health research

While it is undisputed that the framework of medical research ethics cannot be applied to environmental health research just as it is, there is hardly any question about the appropriateness in this context of principlism as such. Very rarely do authors refer to the 'classical' theories of philosophical ethics, such as utilitarian and deontological ethics, but most of them seem to tacitly agree that the approach taken by the Belmont Report is adequate. It should perhaps be briefly mentioned here that Beauchamp and Childress, co-authors of the Belmont Report and the ones who later promoted 'Principles of Biomedical Ethics' not only for research but also for decision-making in the clinics (Beauchamp and Childress, 1979), came from different philosophical backgrounds. The former was a utilitarian, the latter a deontologist, but they realised that if they did not insist on a fundamental approach which would reduce every ethical argument to one and only one ultimate rationale (such as usefulness or individual rights), they could well agree on a number of 'middle-level' principles. These have *prima facie* validity; that is, at first sight they all apply, but they may sometimes be in conflict with each other, which is why in particular situations we have to balance them and argue why one of them should take precedence over the others. In other words, we are not discussing the applicability, relevance, or preference of one over another in general. Instead, we try to make transparent the arguments for and against a certain decision, which may not reflect all principles at the same time to the same degree.

A very similar kind of approach was taken by Soskolne and Sieswerda (1998) when they wrote about the necessity to develop ethics guidelines for professionals in risk sciences, especially environmental epidemiology. At the base of their model are certain aspirations or 'core values' which give rise to 'principles' which, in turn, inform our 'guidelines' and 'standards'. The experience that is gained through research and practice, for example, with 'value conflicts' which may be encountered, will then in a feedback loop promote further evolution of our aspirations. The authors mention the book of Beauchamp and Childress as resource material, but provide no detailed discussion about the 'Principle of Biomedical Ethics' as they might apply in risk sciences.

As to the applicability of the Belmont framework in the context of environmental health research, there does not seem to be much consistency in the literature at first sight. Some emphasise that 'environmental health research does not require new ethical principles, but does require careful attention to the unique challenges it presents for interpreting and applying these principles' (Lavery et al., 2003). Others see a tension between the Belmont Report's 'level of abstraction that allows for flexibility' and 'a desire for greater specification that would allow for more consistent application' (Shore, 2006). Still others simply call for 'A Belmont Reboot', because 'existing frameworks … fit poorly with contemporary research' (Brothers et al., 2019). The latter two studies do not specifically address environmental health research, but have a somewhat broader perspective, referring to community-based participatory research (CBPR). This form of research as applied in environmental health studies is also focused on by Morello-Frosch and Brown (2014), who explicitly speak of 'post-Belmont research ethics'.

All this may look like a trend away from the approach to human-subject-related research established in the late 1970s, but it is clear on closer inspection that the principles are actually not at stake. It is rather their interpretation and application which may have to be re-evaluated in the light of environmental health research carried out over the past decades. If we accept the model of Soskolne and Sieswerda (1998), we should be ready to review even our fundamental aspirations when experience shows them to be lacking, but currently nobody is going that far. Respect for persons, beneficence, and justice are still considered basic, although they may have to be specified differently in the context of contemporary environmental health research, their balance in conflict situations may look differently, and they may have to be complemented with other principles which were not (yet) taken into consideration by the Belmont Report.

As mentioned above, perhaps the most important feature of environmental health research – and of public health research in general – is the fact that it deals with human populations rather than individuals. This is why a number of authors have suggested that the 'Principles of Biomedical Ethics' proposed by Beauchamp and Childress for a clinical context are not sufficient. These are Respect for Autonomy, Non-Maleficence, Beneficence, Justice – very similar, as will be noticed, to the three principles of the Belmont Report. The main difference is that *non-maleficence* is explicitly mentioned, whereas the Belmont Report takes it as an aspect of *beneficence*. Of the publications that suggest additions for population-related health issues, only a few will be mentioned here, none of which specifically addresses research ethics. Coughlin (2008) and Schröder-Bäck et al. (2014), for instance, have written about public health ethics. They suggest that the set of values that Beauchamp and Childress proposed should be taken as a basis but that it should be extended to include Precaution and Solidarity (Coughlin) or Health Maximisation, Efficiency, and Proportionality (Schröder-Bäck). Similarly, the argument has been made that environmental health ethics should take its 'core principles' from Beauchamp and Childress and that it should also include 'additional principles' – Human Dignity, Precaution, Solidarity, and Sustainability – as well as 'procedural principles' – Inclusiveness, Empathy, Accountability, and Transparency (Zölzer, 2017). The first publication of the International Commission on Radiological Protection on the 'Ethical Foundations of the System of Radiological Protection' proposes a somewhat shorter list of 'core values' – Beneficence/Non-Maleficence, Prudence, Justice, and Dignity – and 'procedural values' – Inclusiveness, Accountability, and Transparency (ICRP, 2018). The Commission speaks of 'values' because there are well-established 'principles' of radiological protection (Justification, Optimisation, Dose Limitation), and the Commission wanted to avoid using the same term again.

In what follows, I will discuss different aspects of environmental health research and identify relevant ethical principles and/or core values. At some points, I will come back to the question how much of it is 'Belmont' or 'post-Belmont', and how further progress in research ethics for environmental health can be achieved.

Considerations which apply before research is begun

Naively, one might assume that ethics comes into play when research is actually carried out, or when its results are going to be acted upon. But value-laden decisions have to be made much earlier, when environmental health problems are identified or their existence is suspected. What can be considered sufficient reason to start an investigation – or not to start it? Financial and human resources are always scarce, and not every claim of an untoward health effect can be followed up without weighing its importance against that of other claims – where the term 'importance' itself can have vastly different meanings.

On a general level, we will want to make sure that the question we are about to study is indeed of relevance to public health and that our results can be expected to help reduce health risks (Kass, 2001; Merlo et al., 2007; Schulte and Smith, 2011). Already here, of course, we encounter problems: in order to assess the relevance and impact which our investigation might have we need 'tangible evidence ... rather than media coverage' (Adler, 2004). But 'tangible evidence' is an elastic concept, and does not 'media coverage' often identify problems perceived by the population? Laypeople are the main discoverers of environmental health problems (Brown, 2003; Cordner et al., 2012) and should be taken seriously. Respect for persons demands as much, and so does empathy (Brown, 2003; Wild and Kleinjans, 2003; Zölzer and Zölzer, 2020). Putting ourselves in the shoes of others does not necessarily mean accepting all of their arguments, but it certainly means widening our perspective and admitting that as 'outsiders' to the situation we may be prone to missing important aspects which the 'insiders' could contribute. This may relate to cumulative exposures by different agents versus single-agent exposures (Morello-Frosch and Brown, 2014), or to factors other than physical, chemical, or biological ones, in which case psychological, sociological, or ethnographical investigations need to be included (Brown, 2003).

No evidence should be dismissed just because of pre-existing assumptions or the constraints of a dominant paradigm (Soskolne, 2017). This is also a demand which follows from the precautionary principle: 'When an activity raises threats of harm to human health or the environment, precautionary measures should be taken even if some cause and effect relationships are not fully established scientifically' (Wingspread Conference, 1998). Applied to research ethics, this suggests that investigations should be undertaken if there are threats to human health or the environment even if the evidence so far is inconclusive. Again note that this is usually not taken to mean that any claim to an environmental health problem, no matter how unfounded, should be made the object of research. Some authentic reports, some documented findings, some reasonable assumptions should be available, because otherwise human and financial resources would be wasted which could have been better applied to more serious situations.

Fairness does not necessarily mean treating everybody's requests, demands, or needs equally. As Rawls has argued in his *Theory of Justice*, it may actually admit inequalities, if they are 'arranged ... to the greatest benefit of the least advantaged' (Rawls, 1971). In many cases, it may be ethically demanded to use whatever limited resources are available for the investigation of the problems which confront the least advantaged – or more vulnerable – groups (Soskolne, 1997; Emanuel et al., 2004; Shore, 2006). These may be individuals and groups in developed countries, or on a global scale, whole populations of developing countries (Schulte and Smith, 2011), who are exposed to higher levels of environmental agents influencing human health, have less information available to know about and avoid risks, and also lack political and legal power to change their situation.

A special category of vulnerable people is that of children. They often have higher exposures to chemicals, not least because of their shorter stature; they tend to be more sensitive because they are still in the period of growth and development; and they have longer lives before them in which health effects can become apparent (Ferguson et al., 2017). Although children under the age of 5 make up 12% of the world's population, they account for more than 40% of the environmentally related disease burden (Wild and Kleinjans, 2003). A number of authors have therefore highlighted the importance of collecting age-specific data and of putting special emphasis on children in environmental health studies (Lanphear et al., 2006; Merlo et al., 2007; Sly et al., 2009).

In the context of social justice, the increasingly important role of communities in environmental health research should not go unmentioned. Of course, it is not easy to define the term 'community' to everybody's satisfaction (Cornwall and Jewkes, 1995), and there is scepticism about whether it should be used at all (Adler, 2004). No population that is exposed to certain environmental factors is completely homogeneous. There may be a wide range of experiences, concerns, and expectations which are difficult to describe as those of a particular 'community' (Brown, 2003; Mikesell et al., 2013). It may even be difficult to find out what these experiences, concerns, and expectations are, because we usually do not have access to every individual in a population, but rather to representatives of whom it is not always clear to what extent they really represent the generality of that population (Sharp, 2003; Lavery et al., 2003; Mikesell et al., 2013). Nevertheless, it is clear that underprivileged, vulnerable, and disempowered communities do exist (Coughlin, 1996). Not infrequently, they are communities of indigenous people, or 'island' populations, who are unique not only with respect to the environment they live in but also to social relationships, cultural habits, food preferences, and so on (Shore, 2006; Schulte and Smith, 2011; Cordner et al., 2012). Less well-defined are 'communities of colour', but whatever delineation is used, it is clear that there is a tendency for these to bear a disproportionate burden of environmental health risks (Coughlin, 1996; Weed and McKeown, 2003; Schulte and Smith, 2011). Therefore, thinking in terms of communities can help the implementation of justice when selecting a study population, and in a world in which racial, social, and economic discrimination is still rampant, it can also contribute to a greater consideration of human dignity (Childress et al., 2002; Lavery et al., 2003; Mikesell et al., 2013).

Considerations which apply while research is carried out

Environmental health research can take different forms. In some cases, it may be possible and even reasonable to intentionally expose volunteers to environmental factors. This sounds rather detestable, but certainly much depends on the expected effects: there must be a difference between factors causing allergic reactions and others causing cancer. It has been argued that intentional exposure studies can be ethically justified if they produce net benefit: risks should be minimised, we should be able to gain knowledge that we would not be able to acquire by other methods, and the study participants should receive some compensation, such as medical evaluation (Resnik, 2007). With respect to risk minimisation, however, it seems appropriate to keep in mind the above-mentioned precautionary principle: we should rather err on the side of overestimating the risks (Marchant, 2003; Lavery et al., 2003; Schulte and Smith, 2011), and we should take into account different kinds of risks – medical, psychological, and social (Kass, 2001).

Another kind of environmental health study is where we intervene with exposure in different ways for different parts of the affected population to see how effective certain measures are. Here, we encounter mainly questions of justice: how do we assign people to one or the other branch of our study, and how soon do we share knowledge gained, so that everybody profits (Lanphear et al., 2006; Resnik, 2008)?

By far, the most widely used approach in environmental health research, of course, is epidemiological. It examines correlations between exposures and the occurrence of diseases. In order to do so, it requires detailed and diverse information, not only on particular exposures and particular diseases but also on many other factors which may have an influence on a potential cause–effect relationship. Handling such information can be a highly sensitive issue, and the concept of privacy is much discussed in this context (Childress et al., 2002; Emanuel et al., 2004; Resnik, 2012). It is broadly connected with the principle of respect for persons and has great importance for a trustful relationship between researchers and study participants (Brown, 2003; Weed and McKeown, 2003; Mikesell et al., 2013). We should be aware, however, that perspectives on privacy may not be the same for all stakeholders (Schulte and Smith, 2011) and that there have been significant changes over the past decades (Brothers et al., 2019).

For all three types of research, what is considered fundamental and is not left unmentioned by any author in the field is 'informed consent'. As described above, it is even a pre-Nuremberg concept. That does not mean that it has always been understood in the exact same way or that it might not be 'culturally biased' (Shore, 2006). To say, however, that it reflects 'the near obsession with autonomy in US bioethics' (Emanuel et al., 2000) seems to be going a bit too far. It is widely agreed that study participants should know what kind of research they are involved in, what data will be collected, what risks they might encounter, and so on and that they should freely and without coercion give their consent. It is also agreed that coercion can take different forms, from threats to body and life to economic pressure (Ghooi, 2014).

Particular considerations apply again for children. Generally, proxy consent by the parents is found acceptable, but insufficiencies in the guidelines have been identified (Lanphear et al., 2006). Also, it may be difficult to set fixed rules with respect to age. Youth at the age of 13–16 may be perfectly able to decide for themselves whether they want to participate in a study, or (if they have been recruited at an earlier age), whether they want to continue or to withdraw. It may therefore be necessary to repeatedly ask for informed consent (Merlo et al., 2007).

As concerns research on communities, it is probably common sense that there can never be real 'community consent' (Adler, 2004). The problem of who represents the community was briefly mentioned above. And even when that question is settled, that does not take away from the importance of individual consent. Nevertheless, the proponents of Community-based Participatory Research (CBPR) maintain that the community as such – if a community can be identified – can play an important role in shaping research about their environmental health to make it consent-able. What we are striving for is not any more research 'on' communities but research 'with' communities. Concepts such as 'stakeholder involvement' (Suk and Anderson, 1999), 'popular epidemiology' (Brown, 2003), 'citizen science' (Liutsko et al., this volume), and 'co-expertise' (Lochard, this volume) testify to the shift of focus to participatory methods (Cornwall and Jewkes, 1995).

Of course, it has been rightly stated that 'conducting CBPR does not automatically ensure the ethics of the work' (Mikesell et al., 2013). Things may actually become more challenging because we now have to take into consideration community values and expectations in addition to and together with our own values and expectation as researchers (Mikesell et al., 2013). We need to understand cultural specificities before an acceptable methodology can be worked out (Adler, 2004), which speaks in favour of having ethnographical and sociological co-workers on the team (Brown, 2003). It has been suggested that 'the methods used should be the ones that are best for the community itself' (Shore, 2006), but there is no guarantee that these are the best methods from the scientific point of view (Cordner et al., 2012). The community may be less interested in a methodologically sound study than in advocacy for their worries – which nobody can actually blame them for (Brown, 2003; Sharp, 2003). It cannot be denied that there are such methodological challenges, but then – are we not supposed to show respect for persons, be empathetic with their concerns, include all concerned in the decision-making? If we want both methodically and ethically sound research, we need to get used to 'reflexive research ethics' (Cordner et al., 2012), where researchers are ready to question their traditional approaches and rethink the design, implementation, and evaluation of their research together with the people they study. 'Post-Belmont ethics' does not deny the importance of the principles established for research on human subjects but seeks to promote 'continued reflexivity' and 'a more integrated, and community-engaged perspective' (Morello-Frosch and Brown, 2014).

The International Society for Environmental Epidemiology (ISEE) has published Ethics Guidelines which address many of the points mentioned above, including the Principles of Biomedical Ethics and the Precautionary Principle as well as things like 'accessible language', 'community input', and 'cultural sensitivity of consent'. Altogether, it lists 27 'obligations to individuals and communities', 25 'obligations to society', 5 'obligations to funders/sponsors and employers', and 10 'obligations to colleagues'. There is no space here to discuss these suggestions further, but the document is a must-read for anybody planning research in the field of environmental health (ISEE, 2012).

Considerations which apply after research is completed

There is a debate on what exactly should be part of research ethics once a research project has come to an end and the results have been made available to a scientific audience in the form of conference papers and journal publications. Broad consensus can be noted with respect to feedback by the researcher to the study participants. The assumption that 'they will not want to know,' as the scientific information will have little meaning for laypeople and may even be worrying, is now considered paternalistic and not in line with respect for persons (Weed and McKeown, 2003; Schulte and Smith, 2011; Brothers et al., 2019). Study results should be shared with those whom they immediately concern, but we have to make sure that they understand the disclosed information (National Institute of Health, cited by Shalowitz and Miller, 2005). It is of particular importance to convey an assessment of the uncertainty of our findings (Emanuel et al., 2004; Cordner et al., 2012; Meskens, 2019).

Some thought has been given to findings which may be of immediate consequence for the study participant concerned. Researchers are seen to have 'an ancillary duty of care' (Brothers et al., 2019), which means that incidental findings about health conditions of research participants should be reported back to them (Resnik, 2012) or, in case of children, to their families (Lanphear et al., 2006). Less agreement seems to prevail where the findings concern distributional extremes, especially in biomarker studies regarding the susceptibility to health effects induced by possible future exposures (Soskolne, 1997; Schulte and Smith, 2011; Kalman and Oughton, 2020). It is clear such data should be kept private so that misuse can be prevented; for example, employers should not be able to use the information available for selecting the 'fittest' employees for certain types of work. But beyond that there comes a lack of clarity about the extent to which such results should be made available to the concerned people themselves. On the one hand, they may want to be informed in order to make their own choices, and on the other, they may wish to avail themselves of the 'right to not know' as susceptibility studies cannot provide more than statements on probability, and people may prefer not to burden themselves with worries. In any case, such questions should be anticipated during the design phase of pertinent studies (Schulte and Smith, 2011).

In the case of community research, all of the above considerations apply in a similar way. Research results should be shared even if they are not 'flattering or beneficial' for the community (Mikesell et al., 2013). This could be the case, for instance, if they suggest negative health consequences of traditional ways of life. Keeping uncomfortable results in the drawer is not compatible with respect for persons and the related demands of transparency and accountability (Childress et al, 2002; Shore, 2006; Mikesell et al., 2013). Even in the extreme case where community representatives might push for nondisclosure of certain results, most researchers would not agree – or rather they would have excluded this option from the beginning.

It has to be admitted, however, that the social responsibilities of researchers are not seen by everybody in the same way. Some see advocacy for communities, especially for vulnerable communities, or the empowerment of such communities to self-advocate, as an ethical demand (Weed and McKeown, 2003; Shore, 2006; Cordner et al., 2012). Some argue for less direct involvement but agree that researchers have a role to play beyond the collection and reporting of data and should accompany study participants, in particular participating communities, in their endeavour to understand and interpret research results and to draw conclusions for practice (Schulte and Smith, 2011; Mikesell et al., 2013; Meskens, 2019).

Is all this globally applicable?

By way of a summary, I would like to briefly discuss again the principles underlying all of the considerations outlined above, and the question of their universality. In their seminal book of 1979, which very much echoed the Belmont Report published a few years earlier, Beauchamp and Childress just claimed that the 'Principles of Biomedical Ethics' would be agreeable to 'all morally serious persons' (Beauchamp and Childress, 1979). Later they reworded this to 'all persons committed to morality' and said that the principles were rooted in 'common morality', which is 'not relative to cultures and individuals, because it transcends both' (Beauchamp and Childress, 2013). They expressed scepticism about the possibility to show such universality in empirical studies, and I agree with this assessment. A universal 'opinion poll', which would find out what people around the globe are thinking about the pertinent questions, would just reflect current dispositions and would be very much subject to fluctuations. Something with greater long-term validity is needed. Orientation has been provided throughout the ages by the religious and philosophical traditions of the different cultures (Zölzer, 2017). In my view, the most important documents for establishing a 'common morality' are the sacred scriptures of the world's great religions, which in spite of the declining role of religion in parts of the 'Western' world still provide

Table 12.1 Principles of research ethics

Belmont principle	Additional principle	Procedural principle
Respect for persons		Inclusiveness
Beneficence	Solidarity	Empathy
(including non-maleficence)	Precaution	Accountability
Justice		Transparency

a framework of orientation for many people around the world. There are also relevant cultural expressions outside the context of (organised) religion. Thus, oral traditions in the form of proverbs, stories, legends, and myths, especially those of indigenous people who have no written records, should not be ignored. In addition, secular texts of various types that have had a formative influence over the centuries should be considered. The Hippocratic Oath comes to mind, or the works of certain philosophers of ancient Greece and China (even if Confucius' writings are perhaps more appropriately classified as sacred scripture). In addition to these time-honoured traditions, some modern documents such as the 'Universal Declaration of Human Rights' or the 'Universal Declaration on Bioethics and Human Rights' have been suggested to already constitute 'common heritage of humankind' (ten Have and Gordijn, 2013). In all these traditions, we do find evidence of the basic principles promoted by the Belmont Report (as well as Beauchamp and Childress), and we can also identify further principles which have applicability beyond the context of clinical medicine, namely for public health in general and environmental health in particular. My suggestion was to arrange these principles in a table that gave an overview of core, additional and procedural principles and indicated at least some of their relationships (Zölzer, 2017). This table is reproduced here in a form modified so that the Belmont principles (not the Principles of Biomedical Ethics) are considered core.

Respect for persons is listed first. For clinical medicine, Beauchamp and Childress preferred to narrow it down to 'respect for autonomy', whereas I have argued that in the context of environmental health we should complement it with the broader (and in a way more fundamental) concept of 'human dignity'. That is in agreement with the ICRP's choice of 'core values' for radiological protection (ICRP, 2018). Taking seriously people's dignity can and should be reflected in including them with the assessment of environmental health problems and decision-making about their solution. Inclusiveness can be considered as the key concept behind stakeholder participation.

Beneficence and Non-Maleficence are seen by the Belmont Report (and by ICRP, for that matter) as too closely connected to be separated, but Beauchamp and Childress saw both as distinct principles in their own right. Beneficence for the individual with whom the physician may work is complemented by solidarity which the public health specialist shows to affected populations, especially vulnerable ones. This is closely related to what was discussed above as 'social justice' – giving special attention to the underprivileged. The related procedural value is empathy, which encourages us to see things from the perspective of the other. As a principle or value in environmental health it is relatively unknown, but that seems to be changing.

Non-maleficence urges avoidance of immediate harm done by the doctor to the patient. Extended to larger populations and different kinds of risks, it should be complemented by precaution, which deals with uncertain and not easily quantifiable harms. Because we have to give attention to obvious as well as potential harms, and also have to balance this with the beneficence which is possible to achieve, the most closely related procedural principle seems to be accountability.

Justice in the areas which we have discussed here is almost always understood as distributive justice, a fair distribution of burden and profit between patients or among different groups in society. I suggested that the appropriate complement here would be 'sustainability', which captures the idea of justice for people coming after us, especially future generations. As far as I can see, sustainability or 'intergenerational justice' has so far not played any role in research ethics for environmental health, which is why the above table contains only the comprehensive term *justice*. As it is only fair for people affected by certain environmental factors to be fully informed about what we know of related health risks (and also for future generations to receive information about the heritage that we leave behind for them), transparency is the related procedural principle in this case.

The arrangement of the ten principles in this table does not have to please everybody, of course, and has to be taken with a grain of salt. Many other relationships and cross-references between the individual concepts could be pointed out. My hope when I introduced this concept, and again now with the modified version, is that it will help to keep an overview and to do away with long lists of related terms which (I feel) do not really add to our understanding of the ethical landscape.

A number of authors have maintained that ethical principles may vary between societies and cultures (Childress et al., 2002; Shore, 2006; Brothers et al., 2019) and that harmonisation is needed (Merlo et al., 2007). It is probably true that there can be many nuances in the understanding of concepts such as respect for persons, or justice, or any of the other concepts mentioned above, and that as the world is more and more turning into a global village, we need to better understand these differences. This will only be possible with the help of cross-cultural interaction, a discourse about the meaning and application of the principles on a global scale.

I do maintain that the principles which have been identified after several decades of environmental health research are acceptable everywhere around the world and that our understanding does not depend too much on whether we come from China, or Gambia, or Guatemala, or Czechia. Differences will be encountered when it comes to balancing. As was said above, these principles all have *prima facie* value, but we may think differently about their respective weight in particular situations. Personally, I am confident that with a few more decades of discourse we will develop a global approach even in this respect. We come from different backgrounds and need to talk much more before we understand each other well. This, to me, is another aspect of 'reflexive research ethics' (Cordner et al., 2012): we have to continue and reinforce whatever cross-cultural discourse there may be, to be ever ready to reconsider our current viewpoints, and to look for commonalities rather than dwell on differences.

References

Abrams H.K. (2001) 'A Short History of Occupational Health', *Journal of Public Health Policy*, 22, 34–80.

Adashi E.Y., Walters L.B., Menikoff J.A. (2018) 'The Belmont Report at 40: Reckoning with Time', *American Journal of Public Health*, 108, 1345–1348.

Adler T. (2004) 'Ethics of Environmental Health', *Environmental Health Perspectives*, 112, A988–A990.

Al Khayat M.H. (1997) *Environmental Health. An Islamic Perspective.* Alexandria: World Health Organisation.

Baker S.M., Brawley O.W., Marks L.S. (2005) 'Effects of Untreated Syphilis in the Negro Male, 1932 to 1972: A Closure Comes to the Tuskegee Study, 2004', *Urology*, 65, 1259–1262.

Beauchamp T.L., Childress J.F. (1979, 1994, 2013) *Principles of Biomedical Ethics.* Oxford: Oxford University Press.

Beecher H.K. (1966) 'Ethics and Clinical Research', *New England Journal of Medicine*, 274, 1354–1360.

Brothers K.B., Rivera S.M., Cadigan R.J., Sharp R.R., Goldenberg A.J. (2019) 'A Belmont Reboot: Building a Normative Foundation for Human Research in the 21st Century', *The Journal of Law, Medicine & Ethics : A Journal of the American Society of Law, Medicine & Ethics*, 47, 165–172.

Brown P. (2003) 'Qualitative Methods in Environmental Health Research', *Environmental Health Perspectives*, 111, 1789–1798.

Cave W., Ed. (1940) *Bernardino Ramazzini, De Morbis Artificum Diatriba.* Chicago, IL: University of Chicago Press.

Chadwick E. (1843) *Report on the Sanitary Condition of the Labouring Population of Great Britain. A Supplementary Report on the Results of a Special Inquiry into the Practice of Interment in Towns.* London: Clowes & Sons.

Childress J.F., Faden R.R., Gaare R.D., Gostin L.O., Kahn J., Bonnie R.J., Kass N.E., Mastroianni A.C., Moreno J.D., Nieburg P. (2002) 'Public Health Ethics: Mapping the Terrain', *Journal of Law, Medicine and Ethics*, 30, 170–178.

Cordner A., Ciplet D., Brown P., Morello-Frosch R. (2012) 'Reflexive Research Ethics for Environmental Health and Justice: Academics and Movement-Building', *Social Movement Studies*, 11, 161–176.

Cornwall A., Jewkes R. (1995) 'What Is Participatory Research?', *Social Science and Medicine*, 41, 1667–1676.

Coughlin S.S. (1996) 'Environmental justice: The Role of Epidemiology in Protecting Unempowered Communities from Environmental Hazards', *The Science of the Total Environment*, 184, 67–76.

Coughlin S.S. (2008) 'How Many Principles for Public Health Ethics', *Open Public Health Journal*, 1, 8–16.

Emanuel E.J., Wendler D., Grady C. (2000) 'What makes clinical research ethical?' *JAMA*, 283(20), 2701–2711.

Emanuel E.J., Wendler D., Killen J., Grady C. (2004) 'What Makes Clinical Research in Developing Countries Ethical? The Benchmarks of Ethical Research', *Journal of Infectious Diseases*, 189, 930–937.

Ferguson A., Penney R., Solo-Gabriele H. (2017) 'A Review of the Field on Children's Exposure to Environmental Contaminants: A Risk Assessment Approach', *International Journal of Environmental Research and Public Health*, 14, 265.

Fluss S. (1999) 'How the Declaration of Helsinki Developed', *Good Clinical Practice Journal*, 6, 18–21.

Forrest Weber C.E. (1995) 'Alice Hamilton, M.D., Crusader against Death on the Job', *Traces of Indiana and Midwestern History*, 7, 28–51.

Ghooi R.B. (2014) 'Ensuring that Informed Consent Is Really an Informed Consent: Role of Videography', *Perspectives in Clinical Research*, 5, 3–5.

Hamilton A. (1943) *Exploring the Dangerous Trades: The Autobiography of Alice Hamilton, MD*. Boston, MA: Little and Brown.

Hien W. (2011) 'Public-Health-Praxis braucht Berufsethik. Plädoyer aus historischer Perspektive', *Zeitschrift für Medizinische Ethik*, 57, 173–184.

ICRP – International Commission on Radiological Protection (2018) 'Ethical Foundations of the System of Radiological Protection', ICRP Publication 138, *Annals of the ICRP*, 47, 1–65.

ISEE - International Society for Environmental Epidemiology (2012) *Ethics Guidelines for Environmental Epidemiologists*, online: https://www.iseepi.org/docs/ISEE_Ethics_Guidelines_adopted_april_25_2012-English.pdf [Accessed 28 June 2021].

Kalman C., Oughton D. (2020) 'Ethical Considerations Related to Radiosensitivity and Radiosusceptibility', *International Journal of Radiation Biology*, 96, 340–343.

Kass N.E. (2001) 'An Ethics Framework for Public Health', *American Journal of Public Health*, 91, 1776–1782.

Koelsch F., Zoepfl F., Ed. (1927) *Ulrich Ellenbog, Von den gifftigen Besen Temmpffen vnn Reüchen. Eine gewerbe-hygienische Schrift des XV. Jahrhunderts*. München: Münchner Drucke, 1927.

Lanphear B.P., Paulson J., Beirne S. (2006) 'Trials and Tribulations of Protecting Children from Environmental Hazards', *Environmental Health Perspectives*, 114, 1609–1612.

Lavery J.V., Upshur R.E., Sharp R.R., Hofman K.J. (2003) 'Ethical Issues in International Environmental Health Research', *International Journal of Hygiene and Environmental Health*, 206, 453–463.

Maehle A.H. (2012) ''God's Ethicist': Albert Moll and His Medical Ethics in Theory and Practice', *Medical History*, 56, 217–236.

Malik A.Y., Foster C. (2016) 'The Revised Declaration of Helsinki: Cosmetic or Real Change?', *Journal of the Royal Society of Medicine*, 109, 184–189.

Marchant G.E. (2003) 'From General Policy to Legal Rule: Aspirations and Limitations of the Precautionary Principle', *Environmental Health Perspectives*, 111, 1799–1803.

Merlo D.F., Knudsen L.E., Matusiewicz K., Niebrój L., Vähäkangas K.H. (2007) 'Ethics in Studies on Children and Environmental Health', *Journal of Medical Ethics*, 33, 408–413.

Meskens, G. (2019) 'The Politics of Hypothesis: An Inquiry into the Ethics of Scientific Assessment', in: *Environmental Health Risks – Ethical Aspects*, edited by Zölzer F., Meskens, G. Abingdon: Routledge, pp. 3–16.

Mikesell L., Bromley E., Khodyakov D. (2013) 'Ethical Community-Engaged Research: A Literature Review', *American Journal of Public Health*, 103, e7–e14.

Moll A. (1902) *Ärztliche Ethik; die Pflichten des Arztes in allen Beziehungen seiner Thätigkeit*. Stuttgart: Enke.

Morello-Frosch R., Brown P. (2014) 'Science, Social Justice and Post-Belmont Research Ethics: Implications for Regulation and Environmental Health Science', in: *Routledge Handbook of Science, Technology, and Society*, edited by Kleinman D., Moore K. Abingdon: Routledge, pp. 488–500.

Moreno J.D., Schmidt U., Joffe S. (2017) 'The Nuremberg Code 70 Years Later', *Journal of the American Medical Association*, 318, 795–796.

Müller I., Ed. (2013) *Theophrastus Paracelsus von Hohenheim, Von der Bergsucht oder Bergkranckheiten*. Berlin-Heidelberg: Springer.

Müller R., Milles D., Ed. (1984) *Beiträge zur Geschichte der Arbeiterkrankheiten und der Arbeitsmedizin in Deutschland*. Dortmund: Bundesanstalt für Arbeitsschutz.

Parascandola M., Ed. (2003) 'Ethics in Environmental Health: A Mini-monograph', *Environmental Health Perspectives*, 111, 1786–1818.

Pott, P. (1775) *Chirurgical Observations: Relative to the Cataract, the Polypus of the Nose, the Cancer of the Scrotum, the Different Kinds of Ruptures, and the Mortification of the Toes and Feet*. London: Carnegy.

Rawls J. (1971) *A Theory of Justice*. Cambridge, MA: Harvard University Press.

Resnik D.B. (2007) 'Intentional Exposure Studies of Environmental Agents on Human Subjects: Assessing Benefits and Risks', *Accountability in Research*, 14, 35–55.

Resnik D.B. (2008) Randomized controlled trials in environmental health research: ethical issues. *Journal of Environmental Health*, 70(6), 28–30.

Resnik D.B. (2012) *Environmental Health Ethics*. Cambridge, MA: Cambridge University Press.

Rice T.W. (2008) 'The Historical, Ethical, and Legal Background of Human-Subjects Research', *Respiratory Care*, 53, 1325–1329.

Ringen K. (1979) 'E. Chadwick, the Market Ideology, and Sanitary Reform: On the Nature of the 19th-century Public Health Movement', *International Journal of Health Service*, 9, 107–120.

Schiebelsberger E.M. (2009) *Ludwig Hirt (1844–1907) – Ein Pionier der Arbeitsmedizin*. Doctoral dissertation, University of Regensburg 2009.

Schiffer C., Ed. (1977) *Georgius Agricola, De Re Metallica, Libri XII*. Düsseldorf: VDI-Verlag.

Schröder-Bäck P., Duncan P., Sherlaw W., Brall C., Czabanowska K. (2014) 'Teaching Seven Principles for Public Health Ethics: Towards a Curriculum for a Short Course on Ethics in Public Health Programmes', *BMC Medical Ethics*, 15, 73–82.

Schulte P.A., Smith A. (2011) 'Ethical Issues in Molecular Epidemiologic Research', *IARC Science Publications*, 163, 9–22.

Shalowitz D.I., Miller F.G. (2005) 'Disclosing Individual Results of Clinical Research: Implications of Respect for Participants', *Journal of the American Medical Association*, 294, 737–740.

Sharp R.R. (2003) 'Ethical Issues in Environmental Health Research', *Environmental Health Perspectives*, 111, 1786–1788.

Shore N. (2006) 'Re-Conceptualizing the Belmont Report. A Community-Base Participatory Research Perspective', *Journal of Community Practice*, 14, 5–26.

Sly P.D., Eskenazi B., Pronczuk J., Srám R., Diaz-Barriga F., Machin D.G., Carpenter D.O., Surdu S., Meslin E.M. (2009) 'Ethical Issues in Measuring Biomarkers in Children's Environmental Health', *Environmental Health Perspectives*, 117, 1185–1190.

Soskolne C.L. (1997) 'Ethical, Social, and Legal Issues Surrounding Studies of Susceptible Populations and Individuals', *Environmental Health Perspectives*, 105 Suppl. 4, 837–841.

Soskolne C.L. (2017) 'Global, Regional and Local Ecological Change. Ethical Aspects of Public Health Research and Practice', in: *Ethics of Environmental Health*, edited by Zölzer F., Meskens, G. Abingdon: Routledge, pp. 3–16.

Soskolne C.L., Sieswerda L.E. (1998) 'Implementing Ethics in the Professions: Examples from Environmental Epidemiology', *Science and Engineering Ethics*, 9, 181–190.

Suk W.A., Anderson B.E. (1999) 'A Holistic Approach to Environmental Health Research', *Environmental Health Perspectives*, 107, A338–339.

ten Have H., Gordijn B. (2013) 'Global Bioethics', in: *Compendium and Atlas of Global Bioethics*, edited by ten Have H., Gordijn, B. Dordrecht: Springer, pp. 1–16.

Thackrah C.T. (1821) *An Introductory Discourse*. Leeds: Gawtress and Co.

Thackrah C.T. (1832) *The Effects of Arts, Trades and Professions and of Civic States and Habits of Living on Health and Longevity with Suggestions for Removal of Many of the Agents Which Produce Disease and Shorten the Duration of Life*. London: Longman, Rees, Orme, Brown, Green, & Longman.

Vollmann J., Winau R. (1996) 'Informed Consent in Human Experimentation before the Nuremberg Code', *British Medical Journal*, 313, 1445–1447.

Weed D.L., McKeown R.E. (2003) 'Science and Social Responsibility in Public Health', *Environmental Health Perspectives*, 111, 1804–1808.

Wild C.P., Kleinjans J. (2003) 'Children and Increased Susceptibility to Environmental Carcinogens: Evidence or Empathy?', *Cancer Epidemiology, Biomarkers and Prevention*, 12, 1389–1394.

Wingspread Conference (1998) *Wingspread Statement on the Precautionary Principle*, online: https://www.sehn.org/sehn/wingspread-conference-on-the-precautionary-principle [Accessed 28 June 2021].

Zölzer F. (2017) 'A Common Morality Approach to Environmental Health Ethics', in: *Ethics of Environmental Health*, edited by Zölzer F., Meskens, G. Abingdon: Routledge, pp. 51–68.

Zölzer F., Meskens G., Ed. (2017) *Ethics of Environmental Health*, Abingdon: Routledge.

Zölzer F., Meskens G., Ed. (2019) *Environmental Health Risks – Ethical Aspects*, Abingdon: Routledge.

Zölzer F., Zölzer N. (2020) 'Empathy as an Ethical Principle for Environmental Health', *The Science of the Total Environment*, 705, 135922.

Index

For Product Safety Concerns and Information please contact our EU
representative GPSR@taylorandfrancis.com
Taylor & Francis Verlag GmbH, Kaufingerstraße 24, 80331 München, Germany

www.ingramcontent.com/pod-product-compliance
Lightning Source LLC
Chambersburg PA
CBHW060253220326
41598CB00027B/4084

* 9 7 8 1 0 3 2 1 7 1 8 3 8 *